# ACUTE CARE NURSE PRACTITIONER CERTIFICATION

## Study Question Book

*Second Edition*

*Edited by*

## Sally K. Miller, PhD, APN, FAANP

Associate Professor
Department of Physiologic Nursing
University of Las Vegas School of Nursing
Las Vegas, Nevada

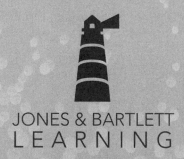

JONES & BARTLETT
LEARNING

*World Headquarters*
Jones & Bartlett Learning
40 Tall Pine Drive
Sudbury, MA 01776
978-443-5000
info@jblearning.com
www.jblearning.com

Jones & Bartlett Learning
Canada
6339 Ormindale Way
Mississauga, Ontario L5V 1J2
Canada

Jones & Bartlett Learning
International
Barb House, Barb Mews
London W6 7PA
United Kingdom

Jones & Bartlett Learning books and products are available through most bookstores and online booksellers. To contact Jones & Bartlett Learning directly, call 800-832-0034, fax 978-443-8000, or visit our website, www.jblearning.com.

Substantial discounts on bulk quantities of Jones & Bartlett Learning publications are available to corporations, professional associations, and other qualified organizations. For details and specific discount information, contact the special sales department at Jones & Bartlett Learning via the above contact information or send an email to specialsales@jblearning.com.

Copyright © 2011 by Jones & Bartlett Learning, LLC

All rights reserved. No part of the material protected by this copyright may be reproduced or utilized in any form, electronic or mechanical, including photocopying, recording, or by any information storage and retrieval system, without written permission from the copyright owner.

The authors, editor, and publisher have made every effort to provide accurate information. However, they are not responsible for errors, omissions, or for any outcomes related to the use of the contents of this book and take no responsibility for the use of the products and procedures described. Treatments and side effects described in this book may not be applicable to all people; likewise, some people may require a dose or experience a side effect that is not described herein. Drugs and medical devices are discussed that may have limited availability controlled by the Food and Drug Administration (FDA) for use only in a research study or clinical trial. Research, clinical practice, and government regulations often change the accepted standard in this field. When consideration is being given to use of any drug in the clinical setting, the health care provider or reader is responsible for determining FDA status of the drug, reading the package insert, and reviewing prescribing information for the most up-to-date recommendations on dose, precautions, and contraindications, and determining the appropriate usage for the product. This is especially important in the case of drugs that are new or seldom used.

## Production Credits

Publisher: Kevin Sullivan
Acquisitions Editor: Amy Sibley
Associate Editor: Patricia Donnelly
Editorial Assistant: Rachel Shuster
Production Editor: Amanda Clerkin
Marketing Manager: Rebecca Wasley

V.P., Manufacturing and Inventory Control: Therese Connell
Composition: DataStream Content Solutions, LLC
Cover Design: Scott Moden
Cover Image: © Hocusfocus/Dreamstime.com
Printing and Binding: Malloy, Inc.
Cover Printing: Malloy, Inc.

To order this product, use ISBN: 978-1-4496-0457-8

**Library of Congress Cataloging-in-Publication Data**
Acute care nurse practitioner certification study question book / [edited by] Sally K. Miller.—2nd ed.
  p. ; cm.
Companion to: Adult nurse practitioner certification review guide / editor, Virginia Layng Millonig. 4th ed. c2005.
Includes bibliographical references and index.
ISBN-13: 978-0-7637-7534-6 (alk. paper)
ISBN-10: 0-7637-7534-7 (alk. paper)
 1. Nurse practitioners—Examinations, questions, etc.  2. Family nursing  Examinations, questions, etc.
3. Nursing—Examinations, questions, etc.  I. Miller, Sally K.  II. Adult nurse practitioner certification review guide.
  [DNLM: 1. Acute Disease—nursing—Examination Questions.  2. Nurse Practitioners—Examination Questions. WY 18.2 A189 2011]
  RT82.8.A38 2005 Suppl.
  610.7306'92—dc22

                                                                            2010009347

6048

Printed in the United States of America
14 13 12 11 10  10 9 8 7 6 5 4 3 2 1

# Contents

# Preface

Previously published by Health Leadership Associates, Jones & Bartlett Learning is pleased to present the Second Edition of the *Acute Care Nurse Practitioner Certification Study Question Book*. This book will further assist the user to be successful in the examination process. It should by no means be the only source used for preparation for the Acute Care Nurse Practitioner Certification examination. It has been developed primarily to enhance your test-taking skills while also integrating the principles (becoming test-wise) of test taking found in the *Test-Taking Strategies and Skills* chapter of the *Adult Nurse Practitioner Certification Review Guide* published by Jones & Bartlett Learning. Content for the examination, based upon the content outline from the ANCC updated in March, 2010, can be found in the *Acute Care Nurse Practitioner Certification Review Course* presented by Fitzgerald Health Education Associates. All review programs and books are meant to provide a comprehensive approach to success in the examination process, building upon a strong academic preparation. They enable the users of these materials to be successful in the test-taking process and reinforce the knowledge base that is critical in the delivery of care in the practice setting. Many individuals feel that taking practice test questions is the most important factor in the certification examination preparation process, yet it is but one strategy to be used in combination with a strong knowledge base. Success in the certification examination area is based upon both excellent test-taking skills and a comprehensive understanding of the content of the examination. As a nurse practitioner seeking certification, it is important to not lose sight of the definition and purpose of certification. "Certification is a process by which nongovernmental agencies or associations confirm that an individual licensed to practice as a professional has met certain predetermined standards specified by that profession for specialty practice." Its purpose is to assure the public that an individual has mastered a body of knowledge and acquired skills in a particular specialty (ANA, 1979).

Inherent in the preparation for certification examinations is rigorous attention to the directives and materials from the certification boards. Content outlines and sample test questions are often provided to examinees prior to the examinations. Specifics for each examination including suggested readings will be provided by the individual testing boards.

This question book has been prepared by board-certified nurse practitioners. The questions have then been reviewed and critiqued by board-certified nurse practitioners (content experts) and a test construction specialist. There are 300 problem-oriented certification board-type multiple-choice questions that are divided according to content area (based upon testing board content outlines), with answers, rationales, and a reference list. Every effort has been made to develop sample questions that are representative of the types of questions that may be found on the certification examinations; however, style and format of the examination may differ. Engaging in the exercise of test taking, an understanding of test-taking strategies, and knowledge in respective content areas can only lead to success.

# Contributors

**Lynn A. Kelso, MSN, RN, ACNP-BC, FCCM, FAANP**
Assistant Professor
College of Nursing
University of Kentucky
Pulmonary/Critical Care Department
A. B. Chandler Medical Center
Lexington, Kentucky

**Ruth M. Kleinpell, PhD, RN, FAAN, FCCM**
Professor
Director, Center for Clinical Research and
    Scholarship
College of Nursing
Rush University
Chicago, Illinois

**Candis Morrison, PhD, CRNP, ACNP**
Hematology/Oncology
School of Medicine
Johns Hopkins University
Baltimore, Maryland

# Instructions for Using the Online Access Code Card

Enclosed within this review guide you will find a printed "access code card" containing an access code providing you access to the new online interactive testing program, JB TestPrep. This program will help you prepare for certification exams, such as the American Nurse Credentialing Center's (ANCC's) certification exam to become a certified nurse practitioner. The online program includes the same multiple choice questions that are printed in this study guide. You can choose a "practice exam" that allows you to see feedback on your response immediately, or a "final exam," which hides your results until you have completed all the questions in the exam. Your overall score on the questions you have answered is also compiled. Here are the instructions on how to access JB TestPrep, the Online Interactive Testing Program:

1. Find the printed access code card bound in to this book.
2. Go to www.JBLearning.com/usecode.
3. Enter in your 10-digit access code, which you can find by scratching off the protective coating on the access code card.
4. Follow the instructions on each screen to set up your account profile and password. Please note: Only select a course coordinator if you have been instructed to do so by an institution or an instructor.
5. Contact Jones & Bartlett Learning technical support if you have any questions:
   Call 800-832-0034
   Visit www.jblearning.com and select "Tech Support"
   Email info@jblearning.com

# 1

# Health Promotion and Risk Assessment for Age Cohort

*Lynn A. Kelso*

## Select one best answer to the following questions.

1. A 53-year-old male is ready for discharge after a three-vessel coronary artery bypass graft (CABG). He has a 43-pack-year history of smoking and has discussed his desire to stop smoking. While implementing patient teaching, the acute care nurse practitioner (ACNP) tells the patient that:

   a. Elimination of cigarettes from the house is essential.
   b. He will experience withdrawal after three days.
   c. He may feel tired and nauseated.
   d. He needs to seek counseling to quit.

2. A 53-year-old female has been on hormone therapy since beginning menopause 2 years ago. She has a family history of osteoporosis and asks about preventive measures. The ACNP should tell her that:

   a. She should take 500 mg of calcium per day.
   b. Walking will help protect bone mass.
   c. She could consider taking alendronate once a week.
   d. Selective estrogen receptor modulators (SERMs) might be a better option for primary prevention of osteoporosis.

3. A 41-year-old married female is evaluated in the emergency department with multiple fractures after a motor vehicle accident. Upon further assessment, three large ecchymotic areas are noted on her upper thighs, and radiology reports three healed fractures of varying ages visible in her upper extremities. The ACNP should:

   a. Report findings to the local authorities.
   b. Discuss the case with a social worker.
   c. Provide her with information about shelters.
   d. Assess the patient for a history of violence.

4. The ACNP is discussing exercise with a 49-year-old male who is concerned about his health status. He states that

he is trying to go to the gym three times a week. The ACNP explains that:

a. Achieving maximal heart rate for 20 minutes, three times a week, is adequate.
b. After the age of 50 exercise does not decrease the risk of heart disease.
c. Optimal goals include both aerobic activity and resistance training.
d. Any exercise that he undertakes will decrease the risk of heart disease.

5. The ACNP is counseling an obese patient regarding the need to lose weight as a general health promotion measure. The patient says, "I know I have to lose 50 lbs, and I know I need to change both my diet and my activity. I put together a 1500 calorie diet from information I found on the Internet, and I am going to begin exercise by walking 30 minutes a day." This patient is in which stage of change according to the transtheoretical model?

a. Precontemplative
b. Contemplative
c. Preparation
d. Action

6. You are doing a health evaluation of a 42-year-old female. She has annual gynecological evaluations and routine dental and eye care. She has no medical problems and a benign family history. She has no record of blood work screening. Based upon current guidelines for health screening you suggest that the patient:

a. Have a cholesterol level drawn
b. Continue her current routine
c. Schedule a baseline electrocardiogram (ECG)
d. Should have liver function tests (LFT)

7. A 64-year-old Korean female is being evaluated for lower back pain. Her past medical history is unremarkable except for premature menopause at age 48.

She is on no medication, and she has a 24-pack-year smoking history. Your initial orders should include:

a. Serum calcium and phosphorus
b. Bone densitometry
c. Serum alkaline phosphatase
d. Magnetic resonance imaging (MRI) of the spine

8. A 57-year-old black male is being assessed preoperatively. He complains of hip pain, urinary frequency, and awakening at night to void. His past medical history is unremarkable. He does not smoke or drink. The ACNP recognizes that this clinical picture is consistent with:

a. Gonococcal urethritis
b. Pyelonephritis
c. Prostate cancer
d. Lower urinary tract infection

9. The ACNP is evaluating a 38-year-old female. She is 6 weeks postpartum with her first child. Her past medical history (PMH) is unremarkable, and her family history includes a maternal grandmother with breast cancer. The patient should be encouraged to:

a. Have a mammogram
b. Avoid estrogen-based contraception
c. Do regular self-breast examinations
d. Only breast feed for 3 months

10. Current United States Preventive Services Task Force (USPSTF) guidelines for depression screening suggest that:

a. All adolescents should be screened for depressive mood or anhedonia at each primary care encounter.
b. All pregnant women should be screened to assess risk for postpartum psychosis.
c. Screening is only indicated when a mechanism exists for treatment.
d. Routine screening is indicated for women of childbearing age but not for men of the same age group.

11. A 42-year-old African-American female is seen for a routine physical examination. During the examination she has no complaints, and her history is benign. For screening purposes the ACNP should order a:

    a. 12-lead ECG
    b. Glaucoma screening
    c. Sigmoidoscopy
    d. Colonoscopy

12. A 21-year-old white male is admitted for a herniorrhaphy. Because you are aware of the leading causes of mortality for this age cohort, the history should include asking this patient about:

    a. Self-testicular examination
    b. Helmet use while biking
    c. Seat belt use
    d. Alcohol intake

13. Examples of primary prevention include all of the following except:

    a. Drug use prevention programs
    b. Annual influenza vaccination
    c. Routine skin assessment
    d. Routine exercise programs

14. A 54-year-old male is hospitalized following a motor vehicle accident (MVA). He has no significant medical history. Based upon the leading cause of cancer morbidity in men, you recommend that he see his primary care physician following discharge for routine evaluation which should include a:

    a. Chest radiograph
    b. Digital prostate exam
    c. Colonoscopy
    d. Fractionated cholesterol panel

15. You are evaluating a 78-year-old male in the emergency department for altered level of consciousness. His daughter says that although he was fine the day before, this is just normal aging and she would like to take him home. The appropriate action for the ACNP would be to:

    a. Discharge the patient to home
    b. Recommend nursing home placement
    c. Admit for a full diagnostic evaluation
    d. Evaluate for elder abuse

# ◼ ANSWERS AND RATIONALE

1. **(c)** The most common manifestations of withdrawal from nicotine include drowsiness, headache, increased appetite, sleep disturbances, and gastrointestinal (GI) complaints. These symptoms will usually begin within 24 hours of smoking cessation. Since it is stated in the stem that the patient has discussed his desire to stop smoking, it is now important that he be made aware of withdrawal symptoms so that he may cope with them effectively. While eliminating cigarettes from the house is desirable, it is not essential and many patients who quit successfully live in a house with other smokers. Similarly, while outcomes may be improved with counseling or some form of cognitive intervention, it is not essential (USDHHS, 2008).

2. **(b)** Weight bearing exercise for 1 hour, 3 times a week, helps to protect bone mass and is a recommended measure for osteoporosis prevention. Recommended calcium intake is 1500 mg/day, not 500 mg/day. Alendronate is used to treat established osteopenia and osteoporosis but is not indicated for prevention. SERMs are an alternative to hormone therapy, but not a better or preferred form of prevention; in any event, drug therapy is not a form of primary prevention (NOF, 2008).

3. **(d)** The patient has physical indicators (fractures in various stages of healing, multiple ecchymoses) consistent with domestic violence; further assessment is indicated. It is premature to report to authorities, and although discussing

the case with a social worker may help you in determining interventions, the best way to begin helping the patient is to establish that there is a history of domestic violence (Burnett, 2009).

4. **(c)** The American College of Sports Medicine (ACSM) and American Heart Association (AHA) guidelines for exercise indicate that optimal regimens for cardiovascular (CV) disease prevention include 30 minutes of moderately intense aerobic exercise at least 5 times weekly or vigorously intense aerobic activity for 20 minutes 2 times weekly along with resistance training. Maximal heart rate is not recommended; target heart rates are a percentage of maximal rate. Exercise is necessary for those older than 50, and while any activity is better than none, "d" is not the best answer of those choices provided; there are daily exercise routines that confer other health benefits (e.g., peripheral arterial disease (PAD) prevention, mood improvement) that do not reduce cardiovascular morbidity and mortality risk (Minn-Lee *et al.*, 2007).

5. **(c)** This patient has taken some action in assembling a diet plan and determining an exercise program; this is the preparation stage. A precontemplative has no plans to implement change in the next 6 months; a contemplative is planning change in the next 6 months. The preparation stage is characterized by being ready to take action or having taken some action, and the action stage occurs when specific, overt modifications have been implemented. A fifth stage not optioned here is the maintenance stage (Prochaska *et al.*, 1998).

6. **(a)** The National Cholesterol Education Program (NCEP) Adult Treatment Panel (ATP III) recommends that all adults have cholesterol screening beginning at age 20. ECG and LFT are not part of routine screening, and her current routine is not acceptable as it does not assess lipid screening (NCEP, 2002).

7. **(b)** Risk factors for the development of osteoporosis include females of Caucasian or Asian descent, early menopause, and therapy with glucocorticoids. Bone mass measurements are sensitive and specific for osteopenia and predict the risk of fractures. Serum calcium and phosphorus levels are normal with osteoporosis, and alkaline phosphatase levels may only be elevated after a fracture (NOF, 2008).

8. **(c)** African-American males have the highest incidence of prostate cancer in the world. Common complaints of advanced stages of prostate cancer include back and hip pain, bladder pain, and perineal or rectal pain. PSA levels are useful to assess for recurrence, for bulk of disease, and may be helpful to detect prostate cancer in asymptomatic patients. With this patient's presentation it is most important that he be further evaluated for prostate cancer. Gonorrhea is less likely in this age group; pyelonephritis is more likely characterized by fever, flank pain, and vomiting; and lower urinary tract infection is not likely to radiate. While any of these disorders might include this symptom presentation, prostate cancer is the most consistent with age, ethnicity, and symptoms, and is the most serious (USDHHS, 2008; McPhee & Papadakis, 2009).

9. **(a)** Women who have their first-term pregnancy after the age of 30 have an increased risk of breast cancer. This risk increases if the first-term pregnancy is after the age of 35. The family history also increases her risk for breast cancer. While recommendations for mammography are evolving, it is accepted that those with a family history and increased risk should have a baseline mammogram. There is no indication that self-breast examination reduces

risk. Avoiding estrogen-based contraception and limiting breast feeding to 3 months does not correlate with better outcomes in high-risk patients (USDHHS, 2008; USPSTF, 2007).

10. **(c)** Screening recommendations for depression are not stratified according to age group and/or gender; screening is only recommended in clinical circumstances in which there is some mechanism for treatment and follow up. Prenatal depression does not predict postpartum psychosis, but may predispose to postpartum depression (USPSTF, 2007).

11. **(b)** It is recommended that African-American women be screened for glaucoma after the age of 40. Caucasian women should be screened after the age of 50. 12-lead ECGs are not recommended as screening tools. Routine screening for colorectal cancer via any method is not routinely recommended until the age of 50; recommendations do change in higher-risk groups USDHHS, 2008; USPSTF, 2007).

12. **(c)** The leading cause of death in white males younger than 24 years of age is MVA, with young adult drivers having the highest rate of motor vehicle fatalities. Young African-American males are seven times more likely to die secondary to homicide than Caucasian or Asian males (USPSTF, 2007).

13. **(c)** Primary prevention includes healthy practices that prevent onset of disease; these include preventative education, exercise, and vaccination. Secondary prevention includes the screening for asymptomatic abnormalities before disease occurs. Skin assessments are secondary prevention, much like blood pressure screenings, cholesterol screenings, Pap smears, and mammography (USPSTF, 2007).

14. **(b)** Prostate cancer is the leading cause of cancer morbidity in men (lung cancer is the leading cause of cancer *mortality*). Colonoscopy may be the best tool for colon cancer screening but this is not universally accepted; regardless, colon cancer is not the leading cause of cancer morbidity in men. Chest radiograph is not a screening tool, and while cholesterol screening is important and should be performed, it is not a cancer-screening mechanism (USDHHS, 2008).

15. **(c)** An abrupt decline in any system or function is always due to some disease. It cannot be attributed to normal aging. In this case, the acute mental status deterioration is most consistent with delirium, which is a general symptom in the elderly of some underlying process. It requires a full diagnostic evaluation (Landefeld *et al.*, 2004).

## ◼ REFERENCES

American Diabetes Association. (2009). Clinical practice recommendations 2009. *Diabetes Care, 2009, 32,* S1–S97.

Burnett, L. B. (2009). Domestic violence. *Emedicine.* Retrieved on January 1, 2010 from http://emedicine.medscape.com/article/805546-overview.

Cooper, D. H., Krainik, A. J., Lubner, S. J., & Reno, H. E. L. (2007). *The Washington manual of medical therapeutics* (32nd ed.). Philadelphia, PA: Lippincott, Williams, & Wilkins.

Fauci, A. S., Braunwald, E., Kasper, D. L., Hauser, S. L., Longo, D. L., Jameson, J. L., & Loscalzo, J. (Eds.). (2008). *Harrison's principles of internal medicine* (17th ed.). New York: McGraw-Hill.

Landefeld, C. S., Palmer, R., Johnson, M. A., & Johnston, C. B. (2004). *Current geriatric diagnosis and treatment.* New York: McGraw-Hill.

McPhee, S. J., & Papadakis, M. A. (Eds.). (2009). *Current medical diagnosis and treatment* (48th ed.). New York: McGraw-Hill.

Min-Lee, I., Pate, R. R., Powell, K. E., Blair, S. N., Franklin, B. A. *et al.* (2007). Physical activity and public health: Recommendations for adults from the American College of Sport Medicine and the American Heart Association. *Circulation, 116,* 1081–1093.

National Cholesterol Education Panel (NCEP). (2002). *Third report of the expert panel on detection, evaluation, and treatment of high blood cholesterol in adults (Adult Treatment Panel III).* Washington, DC: National Institutes of Health (update due Summer 2010).

National Osteoporosis Foundation (NOF). (2008). *Clinicians guide to prevention and treatment of osteoporosis.* Washington, DC: Author.

Prochaska, J. O., & Velicer, W. F. (1998). Behavior change: The transtheoretical model of health behavior change. *American Journal of Health Promotion, 12*(1), 38–48.

Smith, R. A., Cokkinides, V., & Eyre, H. American Cancer Society guidelines for the early detection of cancer, 2006. *CA: A Cancer Journal for Clinicians, 56,* 11–25.

US Department of Health and Human Services (USDHHS). (2008). Quick reference guide for clinicians, "Treating Tobacco Use and Dependence—2008 Update: A Public Health Service Clinical Practice Guideline." Retrieved on December 12, 2009 from http://www.ahrq.gov/path/tobacco.htm.

US Preventive Services Task Force (USPSTF). (2007). *The guide to clinical preventive services: Recommendations of the United States Preventive Services Task Force.* Retrieved on March 9, 2010 from http://www.ahrq.gov. clinic/pocketgd.pdf.

# 2

# Risk Factor Considerations and Prevention

*Lynn A. Kelso*

## Select one best answer to the following questions.

1. A 30-year-old female with a family history of breast cancer presents for a physical examination. When discussing additional risk factors, you ask about:

   a. Whether she performs self-breast examinations
   b. Fluctuations in her weight
   c. Age at menarche
   d. Any previous abortions

2. You are assessing a 23-year-old male who works as a lifeguard. He has three nevi on his upper posterior thorax. They are all symmetrical and dark brown and range in size from 3 mm to 6.3 mm. The next appropriate step would be to:

   a. Question about family history
   b. Teach skin self-evaluation
   c. Refer to dermatology
   d. Instruct him to return in 3 months for follow-up

3. A 45-year-old male is scheduled for a cholecystectomy. He has a history of cholelithiasis and multiple bouts of cholangitis with partial and complete bile duct obstruction. During his pre-operative assessment, he complains of increased bruising and bleeding gums. The next appropriate step would be to order:

   a. Vitamin K 10 mEq SQ
   b. Platelets one 6 pack IV
   c. A CBC, CMP, and coagulation studies
   d. A hematology consult

4. Mrs. Young is scheduled for an elective knee replacement for osteoarthritis. During the evaluation you learn that her past medical history is significant for hypertension, diabetes mellitus (DM), and a myocardial infarction (MI) 4 months ago. The next appropriate step would be to:

   a. Schedule an ECG and echocardiogram
   b. Order a cardiology consult
   c. Postpone surgery for 2 months
   d. Begin treatment with beta adrenergic antagonists preoperatively

5. A 30-year-old female has been in the emergency department three times for fractures that are a result of domestic

violence. Risk assessment must include questions about:

a. Access to firearms
b. Prior drug and/or alcohol abuse
c. History of child abuse
d. Her husband's occupation

6. In accordance with United States Preventive Services Task Force guidelines, all adolescents should be screened at least once with:

a. GC and chlamydia cultures
b. Fractionated cholesterol panel
c. Chest radiograph and fundoscopic exam
d. CBC and urinalysis

7. A 47-year-old house painter is admitted via the emergency department for evaluation of chest pain. He is subsequently ruled out for myocardial infarction, and his diagnosis is pyrosis secondary to GERD. He has not seen a healthcare provider in many years but now expresses an interest in health promotion. You recommend that he begin his routine health screening with:

a. A cholesterol test and tonometry evaluation
b. A digital rectal exam and PSA
c. Stool for occult blood
d. Risk factors for substance-related depression

8. A 62-year-old female presents for a routine physical examination. Her personal and family history is unremarkable for heart disease except for a 36-pack-year tobacco history; however, she states that she stopped smoking at age 48. She asks about her risk for heart disease, and you explain that:

a. Smoking always increases the risk for ischemic heart disease.
b. Once you stop smoking your risk is cut in half.
c. After 10-to-14 years of not smoking there is no increased risk.
d. Risk factors, other than smoking, play a greater role in heart disease.

9. Your 31-year-old patient has a history of splenectomy following traumatic abdominal injuries. Your primary prevention recommendations for her include all of the following except:

a. Mammography
b. Pneumococcal vaccine
c. Always wearing a seat belt
d. Routine cholesterol screening

10. After successfully immunizing a patient against hepatitis B, you expect the serology to show:

a. + HBsAg, + anti-HBc
b. + anti-HBsAg, - anti-HBc
c. + anti-HBeAg, IgG
d. + anti-HBsAg, + anti-HBcAg, + anti-HBeAg

11. A 19-year-old female with human immunodeficiency virus (HIV) is being discharged after a herniorrhaphy. She has a history of asthma. Which factor constitutes an indication for *pneumocystis jiroveci pneumoniae* prophylaxis?

a. A viral load of 5000 copies/mL
b. A CD4+ count of 290 cells/mm$^3$
c. A WBC of < 3,000 cells/mm$^3$
d. Current antiretroviral therapy

12. A 67-year-old female has a history of hypertension, chronic obstructive pulmonary disease (COPD), and Guillain-Barré syndrome. She is allergic to penicillin (PCN) and eggs. She has questions about receiving an influenza vaccine, and the ACNP explains that:

a. An allergy to PCN is a contraindication.
b. Patients with hypertension are at increased risk for influenza.
c. An allergy to eggs is a contraindication.
d. Patients with Guillain-Barré are at increased risk for influenza.

13. When discussing the prevention of sexually transmitted infection (STI) with a 21-year-old patient, the ACNP explains that:

a. Herpes may be transmitted even if there are no visible lesions.
b. Chlamydia is the most common STI.
c. Most STIs have visible symptoms and the risk can be greatly reduced by being aware.
d. Condoms confer significant protection against all STIs.

14. When considering overall risk in the adult patient, the ACNP considers that the most common cause of morbidity and mortality in women is:

a. Coronary artery disease
b. Lung cancer
c. Breast cancer
d. Suicide

## ◘ ANSWERS AND RATIONALE

1. **(c)** Early menarche and late menopause are both considered risk factors for the development of breast cancer due to prolonged estrogen exposure. Self-breast examination is not recommended by the USPS task force for risk reduction. Fluctuations in weight and history of abortion are not linked to breast cancer (McPhee & Papadakis, 2009).

2. **(c)** The warning signs for atypical mole syndrome include asymmetry, border irregularity, color variability, and diameter of greater than 6 mm. Family history is linked to malignant melanoma. This patient should be referred to dermatology for excision and biopsy of the nevi (McPhee & Papadakis, 2009).

3. **(c)** This patient is exhibiting signs that may suggest a bleeding abnormality. Further assessment is indicated to determine whether or not he has an underlying coagulopathy that requires preoperative management. Any intervention is not yet appropriate; further workup is required. If laboratory assessment reveals abnormalities, a hematology consult may be indicated (McPhee & Papadakis, 2009).

4. **(c)** A history of an MI within the past 6 months is a major risk factor for perioperative complications, including acute MI and sudden cardiac death. Elective surgery should be postponed until the patient is at least 6 months post-MI (Fleisher, 2007).

5. **(a)** When assessing the risk factors for escalating violence, there is an increased risk of injury or death in households where there is easy access to a firearm (Fauci, 2008).

6. **(d)** Adolescents only require STI testing if they are sexually active; it is not routinely recommended for all adolescents. Fractionated lipid panels should begin at the age of 20, and chest radiography is not indicated as a screening at all. However, the USPSTF recommends a screening CBC and UA for all adolescents (USPSTS, 2007).

7. **(a)** Fractionated cholesterol screening is recommended beginning at age 20 and then every 5 years. Tonometry should begin at age 40. Prostate screening is not recommended until age 50 unless additional risk factors are present, and depression screening is not routinely recommended (NCEP, 2002).

8. **(c)** The Nurses' Health Study has shown that when a woman stops smoking, one-third of her risk for ischemic heart disease is eliminated within 2 years, and any additional risk was eliminated 10-to-14 years after smoking cessation. Although family history plays a significant role in the development of heart disease, this patient's family history is negative, and so smoking is her only potential risk factor (NHLBI, 2008).

9. **(a)** In the absence of increased risk factors, a 31-year-old woman does not require mammography. However, any 31-year-old should have counseling about seat belt use and accident prevention as accidents are among the

leading causes of mortality in this age group. Similarly, cholesterol screening is recommended for all adults after age 20 due to the risk of heart and vascular disease. Anyone with splenectomy should have pneumococcal vaccination (USPSTS, 2007).

10. **(b)** Patients who have been immunized against hepatitis B will only develop antibodies to the surface antigen, +HBsAg. Those who have natural immunity as a consequence of infection will also demonstrate antibodies to the core (+anti-HBcAg) and antibodies to the core protein (anti-HBeAg) (Cooper, 2007).

11. **(b)** HIV positive patients with CD4$^+$ counts less than 350 cells/mm$^3$ should receive prophylaxis for PJP. Viral load is used as a parameter for changing antiretroviral therapy, but not for beginning prophylaxis. WBC is a general indicator of immune status, but does not guide therapy in HIV. The patient may be on antiretroviral therapy, but if the CD4$^+$ count is greater than 350 cells/mm$^3$, opportunistic prophylaxis is not required (USDHHS, 2007).

12. **(c)** Yearly influenza vaccines should be given to all. There is no contraindication for hypertension or for a PCN allergy; however, an allergy to chicken eggs, or any other components of the vaccine, is a contraindication. While some believe that there is an association between vaccinations and Guillain-Barré syndrome, this has not been established (USPSTF, 2007).

13. **(a)** The only correct statement here is that herpes may be transmitted in the absence of visible lesions due to asymptomatic viral shedding. While chlamydia is the most common bacterial STI, HPV, a viral infection, is much more common. Many STIs are asymptomatic, and it is not possible to assess presence of disease by observation alone. Finally, while condoms do markedly decrease the risk of many STIs when used properly, they do not protect against herpes (CDC, 2006).

14. **(a)** Overall, the leading cause of morbidity and mortality of both men and women in the US is coronary artery disease. Lung cancer is the leading cause of *cancer* deaths, and breast cancer is the leading cause of cancer *morbidity*. Suicide is not among leading causes of death in women (USPSTS, 2007).

## ◘ REFERENCES

Centers for Disease Control and Prevention (CDC). (2006). Sexually transmitted diseases treatment guidelines. *Morbidity and Mortality Weekly Report, 55* (No. RR–11), 1–94.

Cooper, D. H., Krainik, A. J., Lubner, S. J., & Reno, H. E. L. (2007). *The Washington manual of medical therapeutics* (32nd ed.). Philadelphia, PA: Lippincott, Williams, & Wilkins.

Fauci, A. S., Braunwald, E., Kasper, D. L., Hauser, S. L., Longo, D. L., Jameson, J. L., & Loscalzo, J. (Eds.). (2008). *Harrison's principles of internal medicine* (17th ed.). New York: McGraw-Hill.

Fleisher, L. A. *et al.* (ACC/AHA 2007). Guidelines on perioperative cardiovascular evaluation for noncardiac surgery: A report of the American College of Cardiology/American Heart Association Task Force on practice guidelines (Writing Committee to Revise the 2002 Guidelines on Perioperative Cardiovascular Evaluation for Noncardiac Surgery). *Journal of the American College of Cardiology, 50,* 159–242.

McPhee, S. J., & Papadakis, M. A. (Eds.). (2009). *Current medical diagnosis and treatment* (48th ed.). New York: McGraw-Hill.

National Cholesterol Education Panel (NCEP). (2002). *Third report of the expert panel on detection, evaluation, and treatment of high blood cholesterol in adults (Adult Treatment Panel III).* Washington, DC: National Institutes of Health (update due Summer 2010).

National Institute of Heart, Lung, and Blood Institute (NHLBI). (2008). The Nurses' Health Study. Retrieved on December 27, 2009 from http://clinicaltrials.gov/ct2/show/NCT00005152.

United States Department of Health and Human Services (USDHHS). (2007). *Guidelines for the use of antiretroviral agents in HIV-1 infected adults and adolescents*. Washington, DC: Author.

# Dermatologic Disorders

*Candis Morrison*

## Select one best answer to the following questions.

1. A 22-year-old presents with a history of intermittent episodes of red patches on his knees, elbows, and posterior scalp. These are well demarcated and are covered with silvery scales. There is minimal to no itching. What other clinical findings might the ACNP anticipate?

   a. A history of hypersensitivity reactions
   b. Previous exposure to caustic substances
   c. Fatigue, malaise, and low-grade fever
   d. Joint discomfort and Auspitz sign

2. An otherwise healthy patient develops a new rash. He describes it as mildly pruritic. On examination the lesions are oval, fawn colored, and appear to follow lines of cleavage on the trunk. You suspect pityriasis rosea. Which test is indicated in this situation?

   a. Rapid plasma reagin
   b. Throat culture
   c. Lyme titer
   d. Antinuclear antibodies

## Questions 3 and 4 refer to the following scenario.

As the ACNP you are caring for a 24-year-old woman with a history of recurrent urinary tract infections. She was started on prophylactic sulfonamides 2 weeks ago. On day 10 of therapy she became slightly febrile and very fatigued. She then developed circular erythematous lesions from 0.5 cm to 3 cm in size all over her body. Some blistered lesions were evident. The lesions are flat, have pale centers, and are present on her palms and soles. They are nonpruritic. She also developed oral mucosal lesions that now appear as shallow ulcers, and she is having severe dysuria.

3. This clinical picture is consistent with which of the following diagnoses?

   a. Urticaria
   b. Pemphigus vulgaris
   c. Primary syphilis
   d. Stevens-Johnson syndrome

4. The ACNP knows that management of this patient will not include:

   a. Supportive care
   b. Ventilator management

c. IV antibiotics
d. Pain management

5. R. K. is a 72-year-old male who complains of a 3-day history of severe, right sided, lower thoracic pain. Yesterday he began to develop small blisters on the skin over the painful area. On examination, you appreciate grouped, deep-seated vesicles on the posterior trunk at the level of the 10th thoracic vertebra. They stop at the midline. The management of this condition includes:

a. Administration of Zostivax after the acute condition resolves
b. Cephalexin, 50 mg/kg/day for 10 days
c. 1% cortisone ointment bid prn
d. Griseofulvin, 30mg/kg/day for one week

6. A 22-year-old male is seen for a chief complaint of pus draining from his eye. On examination his temperature is 102.2°F. He presents with an acutely erythematous, edematous eyelid and orbit; there is purulent drainage. The ACNP may anticipate a recent history of:

a. Traumatic eye injury
b. Toxic chemical inhalation
c. Acute bacterial rhinosinusitis
d. Sulfonamide use

## ◘ ANSWERS AND RATIONALE

1. **(d)** The combination of red plaques and silvery scales on the elbows and knees with scaliness in the scalp is diagnostic of psoriasis. Psoriasis is a disorder of accelerated dermal turnover, and may have an autoimmune etiology. It is not a problem of hypersensitivity or exposure to irritants, and does not typically produce malaise or fever. It may however be associated with psoriatic arthritis, and Auspitz sign, or the finding of blood droplets when the scale is removed, is consistent with psoriasis (Burns, 2010).

2. **(a)** Though this rash is consistent with pityriasis rosea, a serologic test for syphilis should be performed. Secondary syphilis presents with a macular rash not unlike that of pityriasis. Secondary syphilis may be otherwise asymptomatic at this stage and is readily curable if detected. Therefore, given the potential consequences of undiagnosed syphilis, even though the clinical presentation may be consistent with pityriasis, it is appropriate to rule out secondary syphilis by way of an easy and inexpensive screening test (McPhee & Papadakis, 2009).

3. **(d)** Erythema multiforme is divided into minor and major categories, depending on the degree of mucosal involvement. Erythema multiforme major (Stevens-Johnson syndrome) is defined by systemic toxicity and involvement of two mucosal surfaces (in this case, oral and urethral). It is often associated with drugs; especially sulfonamides, NSAID, and anticonvulsants. Urticaria should be pruritic, and primary syphilis is not characterized by a dermatologic eruption. Pemphigus vulgarus is a blistering disease that is considered "ultra-rare," typically onsets in the fifth or sixth decade, and is not precipitated by drug therapy (McPhee & Papadakis, 2009; Plaza, 2009).

4. **(c)** The treatment of Stevens-Johnson syndrome will not include antibiotics as it is not an infectious disease. Care is primarily supportive, and depending upon the level of oropharyngeal/tracheal involvement, may require ventilator support due to airway edema. These patients also require control of pain and surveillance for secondary infection. Patients with large areas of denuded skin need fluid and electrolyte management (McPhee & Papadakis, 2009).

5. **(a)** This scenario describes a typical case of herpes zoster. Pain follows the course of a nerve and is usually followed in about 48 hours by painful, grouped vesicular lesions. Involvement is unilateral, and lesions are usually on the face or trunk. In immunocompromised patients, generalized life threatening dissemination may occur. While the acute condition will be managed with antivirals—e.g., acyclovir or valacyclovir—management should also include administration of the Zostivax vaccine after the acute episode has resolved. This is not a bacterial infection and is not treated with cephalexin. Similarly it is not a fungal infection, so griseofulvin is not appropriate. Topical steroids are not indicated (CDC, 2006).

6. **(c)** This patient presents with a classic case of orbital cellulitis, often the extension of unresolved acute bacterial rhinosinusitis. This patient needs hospital admission, an ENT consultation, and IV antibiotics. The fever is not consistent with traumatic injury or chemical exposure. Sulfonamide use may produce other consequences, such as Stevens-Johnson syndrome, but not a febrile eye manifestation (Mandell *et al.*, 2005).

## ◘ REFERENCES

Burns, T., Breathnach, S., Cox, N., & Griffiths, C. (2010). *Rook's textbook of dermatology* (8th ed.). Malden, MA: Wiley-Blackwell.

Centers for Disease Control and Prevention (CDC). (2006). Sexually transmitted diseases treatment guidelines. *Morbidity and Mortality Weekly Report, 55,* (No. RR–11), 1–94.

Mandell, G. L., Bennett, J. E., & Dolin, R. (2005). *Principles and practice of infectious diseases,* (6th ed.). London: Churchill Livingstone.

McPhee, S. J., & Papadakis, M. A. (Eds.). (2009). *Current medical diagnosis and treatment* (48th ed.). New York: McGraw-Hill.

Plaza, J. A. (2009). Erythema multiforme. *Emedicine.* Retrieved on January 2, 2010 from http://emedicine.medscape.com/article/1122915-overview.

# 4

# Neurologic Disorders

*Ruth M. Kleinpell*

## Select one best answer to the following questions.

1. A 68-year-old patient presents to the emergency department complaining of profound numbness around his mouth earlier this morning. He first noticed it while brushing his teeth. Shortly after that he became dizzy. His only other complaint was some blurry vision, but he thinks that was due to the dizziness. Symptoms were serious enough to prompt him to come to the emergency department, but they have now resolved completely. Head imaging reveals no acute processes. The ACNP knows that the rest of the diagnostic evaluation should focus upon:

   a. Assessment for neuromuscular disease
   b. Neurogenerative disorders
   c. Diagnostic evaluation for seizure activity
   d. Risk factors for atherosclerotic disease or cardiac emboli

2. Sustained seizure activity for more than 10 minutes may require which management strategies in addition to benzodiazepine administration?

   a. Administration of intravenous corticosteroids
   b. Controlled ventilation to induce respiratory acidosis
   c. Support of blood pressure with intravenous vasopressors
   d. Coma induced via barbiturates or neuromuscular blockade

3. A 32-year-old female presents to the emergency room with sudden onset of left ptosis, diplopia, dysphasia, and left extremity weakness. Edrophium is administered and her symptoms immediately improve. This is because her disorder is characterized by:

   a. An imbalance of neurotransmitters in the CNS
   b. Demylenation of neurons
   c. Autoimmune blockade of acetylcholine receptors
   d. Transient ischemic episodes

4. A 17-year-old male who sustained severe injuries in a motor vehicle accident is being monitored in the ICU. He

develops increased systolic blood pressure, bradycardia, and increased pulse pressure. The ACNP knows that this triad suggests:

   a.   Increased cerebral perfusion pressure
   b.   Direct brain stem compression
   c.   Worsening epidural hematoma
   d.   Critical cerebral hypoxia

5.   A 1-day postoperative craniotomy patient in the neurosurgical ICU begins to develop signs of increasing intracranial pressure (ICP). Which of the following measures would be effective in decreasing ICP?

   a.   Increasing cerebral perfusion pressure
   b.   Decreasing $PaCO_2$
   c.   Increasing mean arterial pressure
   d.   Decreasing $PaO_2$

6.   Ken T., a 16-year-old male, is admitted for suspected meningitis. He has had an elevated temperature of 102°F for the past 24 hours prior to admission and reports a headache with photophobia. Which of the following would be supportive of a diagnosis of viral meningitis?

   a.   Presence of positive Kernig's sign
   b.   Markedly increased protein, glucose, and white blood cell (WBC) levels on lumbar puncture
   c.   Lymphocytes of less than 1000, normal glucose, and normal opening pressure on lumbar puncture
   d.   Markedly elevated cerebrospinal fluid (CSF) pressure

7.   Parkinson's disease is a progressive neurologic disorder characterized by an imbalance between dopamine and acetylcholine. Because of the nature of the imbalance, the majority of drug therapies used in the management of this disease:

   a.   Have anticholinergic side-effects
   b.   Increase natural or synthetic dopamine in the CNS

   c.   May produce bladder spasm, diarrhea, and irritability
   d.   Are contraindicated in patients with dementing disorders

8.   The ACNP is making morning rounds in the medical unit. He awakens his first patient for the day's assessment. While evaluating this 71-year-old patient who is recovering from a hernia repair, he appreciates an acute change in status. The patient is unable to articulate words and has profound right-sided motor weakness. Stat head imaging reveals a significant cerebral infarction. His NIHSS score is 20, blood pressure is 180/108 mm Hg and pulse is 85 bpm. Which of the following precludes the use of thrombolytics?

   a.   The NIHSS score
   b.   His elevated stage 2 blood pressure
   c.   Time of onset of symptoms
   d.   The recent hernia repair

9.   Seizure activity is classified into various categories depending upon symptoms and affected area of the brain. Which of the following is descriptive of simple partial seizures?

   a.   The patient may have aura, staring and automatisms.
   b.   There is no loss of consciousness.
   c.   They are common in children and often involve rapid eye blinking.
   d.   They begin with tonic and progress to clonic contractions.

10.   While managing a patient with pneumococcal meningitis, the ACNP knows that treatment will include:

   a.   Intravenous Vancomycin in all patients except those with GFR less than 30 mL/min
   b.   Antibiotic therapy for at least 7 days
   c.   Dexamethasone in all patients given prior to or with the first dose of antibiotics
   d.   Repeat lumbar puncture after three doses of antibiotic to document sterilization of the cerebrospinal fluid

11. The ACNP is evaluating a 22-year-old male with a chief complaint of profound headache. The patient is holding his head in his hands and says that this is the most painful headache he has ever had. Which of the following additional pieces of information does not support the need for imaging?

    a. Report of a sudden onset of pain
    b. A history of head injury 2 months ago
    c. An absence of any relevant history
    d. Report of associated lacrimal discharge, rhinitis, and rhinorrhea

12. Mr. S. is a 49-year-old male who was admitted 4 days ago for management of a COPD exacerbation. Although respiratory function is improving, he now complains of bilateral lower leg weakness. Physical exam reveals hypoactive deep tendon reflexes (DTR).

    The most likely diagnosis for Mr. S. is:

    a. Rheumatoid arthritis
    b. Myasthenia gravis
    c. Guillain-Barré
    d. Peripheral neuropathy

13. When evaluating headache, the ACNP knows that all of the following except what suggest that the headache is due to a secondary cause?

    a. Age of onset is 52.
    b. There is associated fever.
    c. Pain is "10" on a "1–10" scale.
    d. The pain is worsened with coughing, sneezing, or straining.

14. Ms. Z. is a 23-year-old female who presents to the emergency room with a 2-day history of headache, photophobia, nausea, vomiting, and fever. The differential diagnosis would include:

    a. Pituitary tumor
    b. Viral encephalopathy
    c. Meningitis
    d. Subarachnoid bleed

15. Encephalopathy is suspected in a confused elderly man. Which of the following statements is not correct with regard to encephalopathy?

    a. Hypertensive encephalopathy constitutes a hypertensive emergency.
    b. Encephalopathy is classified as a primary metabolic disease of the central nervous system (CNS).
    c. Cerebral function disturbances result from disease in another organ system.
    d. Encephalopathy is considered an acquired metabolic disease of the CNS.

16. A 28-year-old female presents to the emergency room after being thrown from her bicycle several hours ago. She is alert and oriented, moving all extremities freely, and denies any discomfort. A CT of the head is scheduled. The ACNP notes the presence of ecchymosis over the left mastoid area. This is indicative of:

    a. Fractured sinus bones
    b. Auditory canal hemorrhage
    c. Basilar skull fracture
    d. Epidural hematoma

17. MVA with resultant head trauma is a leading cause of morbidity in young adults, frequently as a function of increased intracranial pressure. What is the mechanism of pressure increase?

    a. Increased CSF volume results in autoregulation and increases ICP.
    b. Increased cerebral perfusion pressure (CPP) produces an increase in ICP.
    c. It increases ICP as a compensatory response to acute volume loss.
    d. The increased intracranial mass due to intracranial edema or hematoma increases pressure.

18. A 43-year-old construction worker is admitted to the trauma unit after sustaining a 40-ft fall. He is intubated but is alert and follows commands. The results of magnetic resonance imaging (MRI) are pending. Upon physical examination, the ACNP finds loss of voluntary movement and proprioception to the left arm and leg, intact loss of pain sensation to the right arm and leg, fracture to the left arm, and suspected spinal cord injury. These findings are most consistent with:

   a. Central cord syndrome
   b. Cauda equina syndrome
   c. Autonomic dysreflexia
   d. Brown-Sequard syndrome

19. Characteristic pain associated with a herniated disk includes all of the following except:

   a. Pain is unaffected by position change and rest.
   b. Pain travels to the buttock or beyond.
   c. Pain is more claudication in nature than radicular.
   d. Associated dermal parasthesias are common.

20. A patient is admitted via the emergency department following an injury during an amateur boxing match. He sustained a direct punch to the forehead, following which he developed upper and lower extremity weakness. Physical exam reveals impaired pain perception and loss of proprioception. Treatment will most likely consist of:

   a. Surgical intervention
   b. Cervical traction
   c. Plasmaphoresis
   d. Steroid administration

## ◘ ANSWERS AND RATIONALE

1. **(d)** This symptom presentation is most consistent with transient ischemic attack characterized by vertebrobasilar symptoms. The patient must be aggressively assessed for atherosclerotic and embolic risk with a goal of optimal control. Neuromuscular disease would not produce these symptoms, but would be characterized primarily by muscular weakness. Degenerative diseases would not be characterized by complete symptom resolution, and while these may be manifestations of some type of seizure activity, the age of the patient and character of symptoms is much more consistent with TIA (Fauci, 2007).

2. **(d)** Sustained seizure activity of more than 10 minutes constitutes status epilepticus. It is considered an emergency state and can lead to hyperthermia, metabolic acidosis, and cardiovascular arrest. Status epilepticus increases cerebral oxygen requirements and increases cerebral blood flow. Parenteral anticonvulsants are used for treatment of seizures; barbiturate coma or general anesthesia with neuromuscular blockade may be required when seizures persist. Steroid use is not indicated. While other disorders may be managed with ventilator induced respiratory acidosis, status epilepticus is not among them. Pressor support is not indicated in the treatment algorithm (Sirven & Waterhouse, 2003).

3. **(c)** These are classic symptoms of myasthenia gravis. The rapid reversal of symptoms when given edrophium is known as the tensilon test. Tensilon is an acetylcholinesterase inhibitor that prolongs enzymatic destruction of acetylcholine (ACh); it is effective because this disorder is characterized by autoimmune-mediated ACh receptor antibodies that block the receptors and inhibit ACh from acting; when given tensilon, ACh lifespan is prolonged and receptor binding is increased (Marino, 2007).

4. **(b)** This clinical triad is known as Cushings reflex and is a sign of direct brain

stem compression that indicates cerebral perfusion pressure is not sufficient to meet oxygen requirements of the brain. This triad represents a response of the cardiovascular system to increase cerebral blood flow (Fauci, 2007).

5. **(b)** Mechanisms to decrease ICP include decreasing $PaCO_2$, increasing $PaO_2$, decreasing cerebral blood flow, and decreasing mean arterial pressure (Marino, 2007).

6. **(c)** Findings suggestive of viral meningitis include some lymphocytes (less than 1000 cell count) but not as much as in bacterial meningitis. Normal glucose suggests the absence of a bacterial population, as does normal opening pressure on lumbar puncture. The presence of a positive Kernig's and Brudzinski's sign are not specific to viral meningitis. Markedly increased protein suggests bacterial infection, as does decreased glucose and CSF with elevated pressure (Fauci, 2007).

7. **(b)** The pathophysiology of Parkinson's disease is that there is a loss of dopamine-producing neurons. Almost all drug therapies seek to replace dopamine, or mimic dopamine, in the caudate nucleus of the CNS. Only one anticholinergic class is indicated for Parkinson's, and is used in those refractory to other treatments. Cholinergic drugs would cause bladder spasms, diarrhea, and irritability—they are not used for Parkinson's disease. Finally, while excesses of dopamine can produce psychosis, appropriate use of dopamine replacement is not contraindicated in dementing disorders (McPhee & Papadakis, 2009).

8. **(c)** The time of symptom onset is the last time that anyone saw the patient acting normally, which for this patient would be the night before. Thrombolytics cannot be used if there has been more than 4.5 hours since

symptom onset. The high NIHSS score is actually an indication for thrombolytics, the blood pressure is not too high (NIH requires SBP < 185 and DBP < 110), and while major surgery would prohibit thrombolytics, a hernia repair is not major surgery (ASA, 2007).

9. **(b)** Simple partial seizures have no loss of consciousness and often involve motor symptoms frequently starting in a single muscle group and spreading to an entire side of the body. Paresthesias, flashing lights, vocalizations, and hallucinations are common manifestations of simple partial seizures. Absence seizures are very brief and occur most often in young children; they are characterized by a brief change in conscious state. (McPhee & Papadakis, 2009).

10. **(c)** All patients with pneumococcal infection should be given a dose of dexamethasone prior to, or concomitant with, the first antibiotic dose. If dose is delayed beyond the start of antibiotic therapy, there is no evidence of improved outcomes. Vancomycin is only recommended when the infection is due to isolates unresponsive to other antibiotic options. Management of pneumococcal meningitis is for a minimum of 10 days, and reassessment of CSF for sterility is not routinely indicated (Tunkel *et al.*, 2004).

11. **(d)** Lacrimal discharge, rhinitis, and rhinorrhea are all consistent with histamine release and are commonly found in cluster headache syndrome; the presence of these symptoms does not require imaging. When the onset is very sudden, this is an ominous finding that does require immediate radiographic assessment. An injury 2 months prior suggests that a subdural hematoma may be expanding. In the absence of any historical information, pain of this magnitude should be imaged (McPhee & Papadakis, 2009).

12. **(c)** Guillain-Barré is an inflammatory process of the nervous system characterized by demyelination of peripheral nerves resulting in progressive, symmetrical, ascending paralysis. Although the cause is unknown, the syndrome often occurs following the exacerbation of a chronic illness. Rheumatoid arthritis is a systemic inflammatory disorder causing arthralgias but not paralysis. Myasthenia gravis presents as weakness in the facial muscles and/or upper extremities, and neuropathy is a sensory disorder without motor involvement (Cooper, 2007).

13. **(c)** The pain of migraine and cluster is frequently described as "10" on a "1–10" scale. However, when the age of onset is younger than 5 years or older than 50, there are associated systemic symptoms such as fever, or the pain is worse with activities that increase intracerebral pressure, a secondary cause is likely (Cooper, 2007).

14. **(c)** Meningitis should be considered in any patient with fever and neurologic symptoms. Acute bacterial meningitis is a medical emergency and prognosis depends on the interval between onset of disease and the initiation of antibiotics (Mandell, 2005).

15. **(b)** Encephalopathy is an acquired or secondary metabolic disease of the nervous system, not a primary problem. When it occurs as the consequence of hypertension, it is considered an emergency requiring intraarterial monitoring and intravenous vasodilation (Fauci, 2007).

16. **(c)** Ecchymosis over the mastoid area, called Battle's sign, is indicative of a basilar skull fracture. Fractured sinus bones tend to present with localized symptoms including face or cheek pain, edema, ecchymoses, or edema. Auditory canal hemorrhage is also consistent with basilar skull fracture, but presents as a hemorrhage in the canal. Epidural hematoma is an arterial bleed that produces rapid mental status deterioration (McPhee & Papadakis, 2009).

17. **(d)** Head trauma increases ICP. As the cranium is a fixed space composed of brain tissue, blood, and CSF, a change in the volume of any one must result in a compensatory change in another. In head trauma, an increase in mass due to cerebral edema or hematoma occurs. Physiologic compensatory mechanisms are transient, and a rise in ICP occurs with head trauma (Marino, 2007).

18. **(d)** Brown-Sequard syndrome is an incomplete spinal cord injury. The injured side displays loss of voluntary movement and proprioception but intact pain sensation, and the opposite side displays voluntary movement and proprioception but loss of pain sensation. Central cord syndrome results from injury to centrally located spinal cord tracts. Movement and sensation may be present in the lower extremities but not in the upper. Cauda equina syndrome results from compression of lower lumbar and sacral roots. Lower extremity paralysis, sensory loss, and bladder and rectal dysfunction can result. Autonomic dysreflexia is characterized primarily by autonomic symptoms such as hypo or hypertension, disturbances in heart rate, headache, and nausea (Cooper, 2007).

19. **(c)** Pain associated with a herniated disk is characteristic and is radicular, virtually always traveling at least to the buttock or beyond; it is not claudication. The pain is not affected by position changes or rest, as is lumbarsacral strain. There is almost always associated paresthesia distributed along the dermatome affected (Hickey, 2009).

20. **(d)** The history of classic hyperextension injury and clinical presentation are consistent with central cord syndrome.

Management centers around steroid administration and monitoring for hypertension and autonomic dysreflexia. Rehabilitation will likely be required after discharge. There is no role for surgical intervention, traction, or plasmaphoresis (Fauci, 2007).

## ◘ REFERENCES

Cooper, D. H., Krainik, A. J., Lubner, S. J., & Reno, H. E. L. (2007). *The Washington manual of medical therapeutics* (32nd ed.). Philadelphia, PA: Lippincott, Williams, & Wilkins.

Fauci, A. S., Braunwald, E., Kasper, D. L., Hauser, S. L., Longo, D. L., Jameson, J. L., & Loscalzo, J. (Eds.). (2008). *Harrison's principles of internal medicine* (17th ed.). New York: McGraw-Hill.

Hickey, J. V. (2009). T*he clinical practice of neurological and neurosurgical nursing* (6th ed.). Philadelphia, PA: Lippincott, Williams, & Wilkins.

Mandell, G. L., Bennett, J. E., & Dolin, R. (2005). *Principles and practice of infectious diseases* (6th ed.). London: Churchill Livingstone.

Marino, P. L. (2007). *The ICU book* (3rd ed.). Philadelphia, PA: Lippincott, Williams, & Wilkins.

Sirven, J. I., & Waterhouse, E. (2003). Management of status epilepticus. *American Family Physician, 68,* 469–476.

Tunkel, A. R., Hartman, B. J., Kaplan, S. L., Kaufman, B. A., Roos, K. L., Scheld, W. M., & Whitley, R. J. (2004). Practice guidelines for the management of bacterial meningitis. *Clinical Infectious Diseases, 39*(9), 1267–1284.

# 5

# Respiratory Disorders

*Lynn A. Kelso*

## Select one best answer to the following questions.

1. A 36-year-old, 72 kg female, intubated for a severe asthma exacerbation, is on the following ventilator settings: Tidal volume ($V_T$) 650 mL; simultaneous intermittent mandatory ventilation (SIMV) rate 14; fraction of inspired oxygen ($FIO_2$) 0.75. Her morning arterial blood gas (ABG) was: pH 7.18; $PaCO_2$ 55 mm Hg; $PaO_2$ 88 mm Hg; $HCO_3^-$ 21 mEq/L. Which of the following orders is appropriate in response to this ABG?

   a. Increase $V_T$ to 700 mL
   b. Increase SIMV rate to 18
   c. Decrease $FIO_2$ to 0.50
   d. Administer 1 amp $NaHCO_3$ IV

2. You are called to evaluate a 22-year-old male who presents to the emergency department secondary to an exacerbation of his asthma. When you arrive the patient is lethargic but oriented. After 1 hour of emergency care he has a BP of 116/82 mm Hg, heart rate 94 bpm, respiratory rate of 24 bpm, and a temperature of 37.2°C. The ABG includes a pH of 7.38, $PaCO_2$ of 42 mm Hg, and $PaO_2$ of 82 mm Hg on 4L $O_2$ via nasal cannula. The most appropriate action would be to:

   a. Admit to the ICU and begin a magnesium sulfate drip in addition to current rescue therapies
   b. Prepare for intubation as his presentation is consistent with impending respiratory failure
   c. Administer inhaled cromolyn sulfate, albuterol, and reassess in 60 minutes
   d. Admit to the floor, begin intravenous corticosteroids, and increase oxygen support to 100% nonrebreather

3. Pulmonary function testing reveals that the patient has stage II COPD. The ACNP knows that treatment should include which of the following?

   a. Short-acting bronchodilators
   b. Inhaled corticosteroids
   c. Long-acting bronchodilators
   d. Nighttime oxygen therapy

4. The patient's chest radiograph reveals an increased retrosternal airspace and flattened diaphragm. The ACNP

accurately interprets this as radiographic evidence of:

a. Acute respiratory distress syndrome
b. Pulmonary embolism
c. Asthma
d. COPD

5. Pulmonary function assessment of chronic bronchitis is the same as that of emphysema. Which of the following assessment/diagnostic findings is associated with chronic bronchitis but not emphysema?

a. Polycythemia
b. Respiratory acidosis
c. Hypochloremia
d. Increased AP diameter

6. Acute exacerbations of chronic bronchitis are characterized by:

a. Purulent mucus production, hypercapnia, and hypoxemia
b. Worsening of baseline dyspnea, cough, or sputum production
c. Fatigue, activity intolerance, and pleuritic chest pain
d. Purulent cough, dyspnea, and hypercapnia.

7. A 72-year-old patient is seen in the emergency department for evaluation of fever of 101.2°F x 2 days and new onset confusion. Her vital signs are as follows: BP 92/64 mm Hg; heart rate 121 bpm; and respiration 26 bpm. Her oxygen saturation ($SaO_2$) is 94% on 4L $O_2$ via nasal cannula. A chest radiograph is significant for a right-lower lobe infiltrate. The patient is diagnosed with community-acquired pneumonia. Which of the patient's characteristics suggest that hospitalization is indicated?

a. Blood pressure and respiratory rate
b. Heart rate and radiographic findings
c. Age and mental status
d. Oxygen saturation and duration of symptoms

8. A patient being treated with IV antibiotics for management of pneumonia develops a large pleural effusion seen on the chest radiograph. A diagnostic thoracentesis reveals clear, pale yellow fluid with a pH of 7.32, protein of 8 gm/dL, and lactic dehydrogenase (LDH) of 1924 IU/L. The ACNP knows that this effusion is best characterized as a(n):

a. Transudate
b. Exudate
c. Chyliform effusion
d. Hemorrhagic effusion

9. A 43-year-old female reports a dry persistent cough. History reveals that she works as a correctional officer in the local county jail where pulmonary tuberculosis has been diagnosed. Her PPD produces 10 mm induration, and subsequent examination of sputum reveals acid-fast bacilli. The next step in her management includes:

a. Isoniazid (INH), rifampin
b. Respiratory isolation
c. Culture and sensitivity reporting of sputum
d. Liver function and visual acuity testing

10. A 64-year-old patient has been on your service for 2 weeks. She was admitted for open reduction of hip fracture, but her hospitalization has been complicated by postoperative emboli. While rounding today, you appreciate a new onset fever. Chest radiograph reveals multifocal airspace consolidation, and her oxygen saturation on 50% mask is 92%. A WBC differential demonstrates 90% neutrophils, and she is diagnosed with hospital-acquired pneumonia. Antibiotic therapy must cover:

a. *Candida albicans*
b. *Pseudomonas aeruginosa*
c. *Enterococcus*
d. *Staphylococcus aureus*

11. Upon admission a patient's ABG reveals a pH of 7.36, $PaCO_2$ of 59 mm Hg, $PaO_2$ of 49 mm Hg, and $HCO_3^-$ of 29 mEq/L on 2L $O_2$ via nasal cannula. The patient is anxious and sitting on the edge of the

bed. He has circumoral cyanosis, and lung fields auscultate for expiratory wheezes bilaterally. The ACNP should order:

a. Lorazepam 2 mg IV
b. Albuterol 2 puffs q2-4h
c. Prednisone 60 mg q6h
d. 60% $O_2$ via face mask

12. A 48-year-old female is in the ICU with acute pancreatitis. Her vital signs are as follows: BP 92/60 mm Hg; heart rate 116 bpm; central venous pressure (CVP) 9 mm Hg; pulmonary artery pressure (PAP) 29/18 mm Hg; pulmonary capillary wedge pressure (PCWP) 14 mm Hg. She is intubated with current ventilator settings of $V_T$ 800 mL, assist control (AC) rate 14 bpm, $FiO_2$ 0.85, and positive end expiratory pressure (PEEP) 5.0 cm $H_2O$. Her ABG reveals a pH of 7.31, $PaCO_2$ of 48 mm Hg, and a $PaO_2$ of 62 mm Hg. Her chest radiograph shows diffuse, fluffy infiltrates.

Based upon this assessment the ACNP would order:

a. An increase of $FiO_2$ to 0.95
b. An increase of PEEP to 7.5 cm $H_2O$
c. An increase of rate to 18 bpm
d. An increase of $V_T$ to 900 mL

13. Recommended ventilator settings for managing a patient with acute respiratory distress syndrome would include:

a. Pressure-control ventilation and a $V_T$ to 800 mL
b. Volume-control ventilation and PEEP of 10 cm $H_2O$
c. Paralyzing and sedating the patient, PEEP of 7.5 cm $H_2O$, and $V_T$ of 6 mg/kg
d. $FIO_2$ of 1.00 and rate of 16 bpm

14. A 21-year-old male is admitted with dyspnea and left-sided chest pain that woke him during the night. He has been experiencing the same pain for 48 hours and sought medical attention because he was unable to complete basketball practice. The diagnostic test that would be most helpful in this situation is a(n):

a. ECG
b. Chest radiograph
c. Echocardiogram
d. Chest CT scan

15. When evaluating a patient with pneumothorax, the ACNP may anticipate all of the following assessment findings except:

a. Hypercapnia
b. Hyperresonance to percussion
c. Pleuritic chest pain
d. Tracheal deviation

16. The ACNP is called to evaluate a 42-year-old male patient for acute onset dyspnea and chest pain. He is on no medications, and his medical history is noncontributory. His only significant social history includes frequent air travel, including a 14-hour trip from Australia late last week. Additional assessment findings might include:

a. A $PaO_2$ of 62 and $PaCO_2$ of 27
b. Convex ST elevations in leads $V_1$-$V_6$
c. Chest radiograph with RML infiltrate
d. Temperature of more than 102°F and hemptosis

17. A 5 mm induration response to PPD testing is considered positive in patients who:

a. Have relatives with TB
b. Live in a community setting such as a military barracks
c. Are on corticosteroid therapy
d. Are healthcare workers

18. A 23-year-old male is admitted with shortness of breath, hemoptysis, and fever. His temp is 38.3°C, BP 116/84 mm Hg, heart rate 108 bpm, and respiration 20 bpm. His chest radiograph shows a left-upper lobe infiltrate.

Admission orders should include which of the following?

a. Sputum gram stain on admission
b. Respiratory isolation
c. Oral corticosteroids
d. IV antibiotics

19. A diagnostic thoracentesis should be performed on all inpatients with:

a. Pneumonia with suspected underlying malignancy
b. Congestive heart failure with effusion
c. Congestive heart failure not responsive to diuresis
d. Pneumonia and coincident effusion

20. The treatment of choice for pulmonary embolism is anticoagulation with heparin. The ACNP knows that low molecular weight heparin is appropriate in all of the following patients except those:

a. Who have nonmassive embolism
b. For whom thrombolytics are being considered
c. Who have stage 3 chronic kidney disease
d. Who are obese

## ◘ ANSWERS AND RATIONALE

1. **(d)** Asthmatic patients who require intubation for severe exacerbation should be treated with IV sodium bicarbonate for respiratory acidosis. Permissive hypercapnia is the recommended ventilatory strategy; however, when pH falls below 7.25, buffering agents should be administered. The goal is to provide adequate oxygenation for the patient, while minimizing high airway pressures and consequently the risk of barotraumas, and while maintaining a pH that is consistent with the maintenance of extrapulmonary function (NAEPP, 2007).

2. **(b)** This patient evidences impending respiratory failure with his rising $PaCO_2$, lethargy, and near-normal respiratory rate. Per EPR-3 guidelines, intubation should not be delayed when it is deemed necessary. Respiratory drive is typically increased with asthma exacerbations, so tachypnea and hypocapnia are expected; a normal $PaCO_2$ and respiratory rate indicate an increased risk of respiratory failure. Magnesium sulfate may delay the need for intubation, but once it is apparent it should not be postponed (Cooper, 2007).

3. **(c)** Stage II COPD requires the institution of daily long-acting bronchodilators such as tiotropium bromide and pulmonary rehabilitation. Short-acting bronchodilators on a prn basis are indicated for stage I, inhaled corticosteroids are added in stage III, and oxygen therapy is introduced in stage IV per World Health Organization GOLDCOPD guidelines (WHO, 2009).

4. **(d)** This presentation is consistent with the chronic alveolar distention of COPD. ARDS reveals a "white" radiograph as alveolar expansion is very limited. Emboli may be apparent as gray or white areas on the radiograph, but not increased airspace. Asthma does not typically alter a normal radiographic picture (Cooper, 2007).

5. **(a)** Chronic bronchitis and emphysema are two conditions resulting in chronic obstructive manifestations and chronic $CO_2$ retention. As a result, both conditions cause respiratory acidosis, with resultant metabolic retention of $HCO_3$ as a buffer; consequently Cl- is excreted, so both conditions will produce hypochloremia. However, because chronic bronchitis is a disease of excess mucus production, patients are trying to ventilate against increased mucus in the airway. They become hypoxemic, and compensatory red blood cell production is increased, resulting in polycythemia. Conversely, emphysema is not characterized by excess mucus production and hypoxemia, so polycythemia is not a common feature. As emphysema is a condition of alveolar distention and loss of elastic recoil, air trapping

produces the increased AP diameter not routinely appreciated in chronic bronchitis. Many patients have features of both, but one form often dominates (McPhee & Papadakis, 2009).

6. **(b)** Acute exacerbations of chronic bronchitis (AECB) by definition are characterized by a worsening in any one of the three cardinal symptoms; dyspnea, cough, or mucus production. All COPD, exacerbation or not, is characterized by hypercapnia, and exacerbations may or may not be characterized by hypoxemia, fatigue, or any of the other symptoms described in the remaining answer options (WHO, 2009).

7. **(c)** In accordance with CURB-65 criteria, a patient who has two or more of five features should be hospitalized for treatment of community-acquired pneumonia: **C**onfusion, **U**remia (BUN greater than 19), **R**espiratory rate greater than 30, **B**lood pressure less than 90 mm Hg, age older than **65**. This patient is confused and more than 65 years of age. While her oxygen saturation and other findings may be considered, CURB-65 criteria specifically indicate hospitalization as appropriate based upon these two of five findings (ATS, 2005).

8. **(b)** A transudate is an effusion that is mostly water, containing little protein, LDH, or other plasma/serum components. When pleural fluid LDH is more than two-thirds, the upper limits of normal serum LDH (333 IU/L), or pleural fluid protein is more than 60% serum protein, the effusion is exudative and suggests a sicker patient. A chyliform effusion is characterized by lipid content, and a hemorrhagic effusion contains blood (McPhee & Papadakis, 2009).

9. **(d)** The presence of acid-fast bacilli warrants immediate management for pulmonary tuberculosis. Liver function and visual acuity tests are immediately performed, and then a full regimen for pulmonary TB is instituted in accordance with CDC guidelines. While culture and sensitivity testing will be obtained, treatment should not be delayed pending results. Respiratory isolation is not necessary in the community setting, and INH and rifampin may be components of management, but they do not constitute a complete regimen; regimens will include a minimum of three agents (Fauci, 2007).

10. **(b)** The patient's clinical course suggests hospital-acquired pneumonia. Absent culture and sensitivity testing, antibiotic therapy should be ordered to cover the same pathogens as those of CAP but must also include coverage for pseudomonas. Additionally, the prolonged hospitalization and character of radiographic assessment support pseudomonal infection (ATS, 2005).

11. **(d)** Oxygen should be administered in order to keep the $PaO_2$ between 55 and 65 mm Hg. This should be done despite the possibility of hypercapnia. Although albuterol would be appropriate, the dose given in the response is not adequate for an exacerbation. Given the respiratory failure, the priority of care here is oxygenation. Once oxygen therapy has begun, an investigation in to the cause of hypoxemia will be initiated (Marino, 2007).

12. **(b)** This patient is at risk for developing ARDS secondary to her pancreatitis. Because of her low filling pressures, it is not likely that she is experiencing cardiogenic pulmonary edema. In order to improve oxygenation, increasing PEEP is most beneficial. Increasing the $FIO_2$ will increase the risk of oxygen toxicity, and you will gain no oxygenation benefit from increasing the rate or the tidal volume (Marino, 2007).

13. **(c)** ARDS requires low tidal volumes and PEEP. Higher tidal volumes and $FiO_2$ are potentially toxic and confer no benefit. There is a need to decrease peak inspiratory pressures, which is best accomplished by using a pressure-control ventilation mode. This sets a maximal pressure limit and also delivers an adequate tidal volume. However, the tidal volumes included in that answer choice are too high. The best combination of those provided is in "c" (Marino, 2007).

14. **(b)** This patient has indications of a spontaneous pneumothorax. Patients are usually young, and the acute onset of ipsilateral chest pain and dyspnea is often of several days duration by the time medical attention is sought. The most important diagnostic examination would be a chest radiograph, which would show evidence of air in the pleural space (Cooper, 2007).

15. **(a)** Increased air and pressure in the pleural space will often result in pleuritic, nonradiating chest pain, and hyperresonance to percussion. More profound pneumothoraces will result in such a pressure increase that the trachea is displaced to the unaffected side. However, hypercapnia, a consequence of hypoventilation, is not expected. Conversely, the decreased oxygenation may produce tachypnea and hypocapnia (Cooper, 2007).

16. **(a)** The symptoms and history are most consistent with pulmonary embolus; the ACNP would expect hypoxemia and hypocapnia by arterial blood gas. The ST segment abnormalities are consistent with anterior wall MI, which is less likely given the absence of a history and the highlight on recent air travel. The chest radiograph would be consistent with pneumonia, which is less likely to produce dyspnea, and while hemoptysis is consistent with pulmonary embolus, fever is not (Kamangar, 2009; McPhee & Papadakis, 2009).

17. **(c)** Patients who may have impaired immune responses are considered positive at 5 mm, such as those on corticosteroids and those with HIV. People who have close contacts with TB patients are also positive at 5 mm, but having a family member may or may not fall into that category. People living in communal settings and healthcare workers are positive at 10 mm (Mandell, 2005).

18. **(b)** This patient has symptoms suggestive of tuberculosis. Patients who are admitted to the hospital with symptoms that may indicate tuberculosis should be placed on respiratory isolation until tuberculosis is ruled out. A sputum gram stain is not adequate, and a sputum for acid-fast bacilli (AFB) needs to be ordered. This patient has no indications for steroids. Antituberculin therapy will be initiated in accordance with CDC recommendations if the acid-fast bacilli are present (Mandell, 2005).

19. **(d)** Any patient being managed in the inpatient setting who has pneumonia and coincident effusion requires a diagnostic thoracentesis. While pneumonia may be the first symptom of an expanding malignant process, a thoracentesis is not indicated if there is no effusion. Patients with CHF do not typically require diagnostic thoracentesis, although a therapeutic one may be indicated if there is no response to diuresis (ATS, 2005; McPhee & Papadakis, 2009).

20. **(b)** Low molecular weight heparin has several advantages over unfractionated IV heparin. It is the preferred form of heparin administration in those with nonmassive PE as long as there are no concerns about SQ absorption. Patients for whom thrombolytics are being considered should not receive SQ LMW heparin because of its long duration of action; the aPTT must be within normal

parameters before thrombolytics are started, and heparin should not be co-administered. If a decision is made to use thrombolytics, the UFH infusion will be discontinued and aPTT normalized (ACCP, 2004).

# ◘ REFERENCES

American College of Chest Physicians (ACCP). (2004). The seventh ACCP conference on antithrombotic and thrombolytic therapy. *Chest, 126,* 163S–696S.

American Thoracic Society, Infectious Diseases Society of America. (2005). Guidelines for the management of adults with hospital-acquired, ventilator-associated, and healthcare-associated pneumonia. *American Journal of Respiratory and Critical Care Medicine, 171,* 388–416.

Cooper, D. H., Krainik, A. J., Lubner, S. J., & Reno, H. E. L. (2007). *The Washington manual of medical therapeutics* (32nd ed.). Philadelphia, PA: Lippincott, Williams, & Wilkins.

Fauci, A. S., Braunwald, E., Kasper, D. L., Hauser, S. L., Longo, D. L., Jameson, J. L., & Loscalzo, J. (Eds.). (2008). *Harrison's principles of internal medicine* (17th ed.). New York: McGraw-Hill.

Kamangar, N. (2009). Pulmonary embolism: Treatment and medication. *Emedicine.* Retrieved on December 5, 2009 from http://emedicine.medscape.com/article/300901-treatment.

Mandell, G. L., Bennett, J. E., & Dolin, R. (2005). *Principles and practice of infectious diseases,* (6th ed.). London: Churchill Livingstone.

Marino, P. L. (2007). *The ICU book* (3rd ed.). Philadelphia, PA: Lippincott, Williams, & Wilkins.

National Asthma Education and Prevention Program (NAEPP). (2007). *Expert panel report 3: Guidelines for the diagnosis and management of asthma.* Washington, DC: National Institutes of Health.

World Health Organization (WHO). (2009). *Global strategy for the diagnosis, management, and prevention of chronic obstructive pulmonary disease.* Retrieved on January 2, 2010 from http://www.goldcopd.org/Guidelineitem.asp?l1=2&l2=1&intId=2003.

# 6

# Cardiovascular Disorders

*Candis Morrison*

## Select one best answer to the following questions.

1. A 62-year-old male presents with complaints of lightheadedness and fatigue of 20 minutes duration. He reports similar episodes occurring over the past 2 weeks. On examination he is slightly anxious. Vital signs are as follows: temperature 36.5°C, heart rate 50 bpm, respiration 18 bpm, and BP 100/80 mm Hg. The chest is clear to auscultation. ECG analysis shows no discrete P waves and irregular atrial activity of more than 350 bpm. Ventricular rate is irregular; however, no ventricular ectopic beats are noted. This rhythm is confirmed in multiple leads. This clinical picture is most consistent with which rhythm?

   a. Atrial flutter
   b. Atrial fibrillation
   c. Ventricular fibrillation
   d. Ventricular ectopy

2. A patient is found to be in atrial fibrillation of indeterminate duration. The immediate treatment goals for this patient include:

   a. Control of the atrial rate and thrombolytic therapy
   b. Decreased cardiac output and anxiolytic therapy
   c. Increased coronary artery perfusion and decreased oxygen demand
   d. Increased atrio-ventricular (AV) node conduction and decreased international ratio (INR)

3. A 64-year-old male is brought into the emergency department with a chief complaint of substernal chest pressure for the past 30 minutes. This is associated with nausea and diaphoresis. He has a history of angina, which was previously relieved with nitroglycerin (NTG). He is a 30-pack-year smoker. He has had three tablets of sublingual (SL) NTG, but the pain persists. Physical examination reveals a heart rate of 80 bpm, respiration of 30 bpm, and BP of 104/60 mm Hg. The ECG demonstrates ST segment elevation in leads II, III, and aVF. Based on these symptoms and findings, the ACNP knows that the _____ wall of the heart is affected.

*(handwritten: II III AVF = Inferior)*

a. Anterior
b. Lateral
c. Posterior
d. Inferior

4. When considering the initiation of thrombolytic therapy in acute coronary syndrome, the ACNP knows that which of the following would be a contraindication?

   a. Age of 72 years
   b. SBP of 160/88 mm Hg
   c. Absence of confirming enzymes
   d. T wave inversion in leads II, III and aVF

5. A 79-year-old postacute MI patient has been in the CCU for 3 days. She now reports constant pain that worsens with deep inspiration. She says she is most comfortable leaning forward in her bed. Vital signs include a heart rate of 112 bpm, respiration of 24 bpm, and BP of 130/79 mm Hg. The ACNP might expect which of the following additional assessment findings?

   a. A $PaO_2$ < 70 mm Hg on ABG
   b. ST elevations in leads $V_1$–$V_6$
   c. JVD 5 cm above the clavicle
   d. Pericardial friction rub to auscultation *(handwritten: = pericarditis)*

6. A patient presents to the emergency department complaining of sharp, stabbing chest pains right over his heart; he is afraid he is having a heart attack. Physical examination is normal, and ECG reveals concave ST-T wave elevations in 11 of 12 leads. The ACNP knows that this condition is best managed with:

   a. SL NTG
   b. Beta adrenergic antagonists
   c. Calcium channel antagonists
   d. NSAIDs

7. An 88-year-old patient is admitted from the nursing home in acute congestive heart failure (CHF). Nursing home staff reports that his normal weight is 71 kg. Upon admission his vital signs include a heart rate of 104 bpm, respiration of 28 bpm, and BP of 120/60 mm Hg. His weight is 73.5 kg. Cardiovascular examination reveals regular rate and rhythm. There are crackles in both lung bases. After several hours in the intensive care unit, he becomes increasingly short of breath and you hear an $S_3$ at the apex. His BP has decreased to 80/60 mm Hg and his heart rate has risen to 130 bpm. He is breathing 40 times per minute. Your immediate treatment goals are to:

   a. Reduce preload and afterload
   b. Reduce afterload and contractility
   c. Reduce preload and improve contractility
   d. Reduce afterload and improve contractility

8. Assessment findings in the patient with chronic congestive heart failure would include all of the following except:

   a. Diffuse chest wall heave and JVD
   b. Redistribution of flow on chest radiograph
   c. Abdominal discomfort and venous hum
   d. Diffuse rales to auscultation and $S_3$ heart sound

9. While performing a preoperative H&P on a patient, the ACNP appreciates a systolic murmur at the second intercostal space, right sternal border. This is consistent with which of the following types of murmurs?

   a. Aortic stenosis
   b. Pulmonic regurgitation
   c. Mitral regurgitation
   d. Pulmonary stenosis

10. Many critical care units typically monitor a patient's heart rate and rhythm in lead II. This is an example of:

    a. Traditional practice
    b. Evidence-based practice
    c. Cost-effective practice
    d. USPS Task Force recommended practice

11. The ACNP is evaluating a patient who complains of intermittent pain at rest and paresthesia in the right-lower extremity. His history is significant for coronary artery disease and hypertension that is well controlled on beta adrenergic blockade. Physical examination reveals that the right leg has 1+ edema, is cold to palpation, pale, and has diminished hair growth. The appropriate intervention will likely include:

    a. Aggressive revascularization measures
    b. Anticoagulation
    c. Compression stockings
    d. Walking to the point of pain followed by rest

12. A patient has been admitted for the evaluation of progressive shortness of breath with everyday activity and episodes of vertigo. The history reveals use of fen-phen for weight loss, and a diagnostic evaluation is begun to rule out pulmonary hypertension. Which of the following assessment findings is not consistent with pulmonary hypertension?

    a. A hilar/thoracic ratio > 0.44 on chest radiograph
    b. Tricuspid regurgitation on chest radiograph
    c. An R/S ratio > 0.5 in $V_1$
    d. Right ventricular dilation

13. A 60-year-old patient is brought to the emergency department with a history of severe substernal chest pain. It has not been relieved with three doses of nitroglycerin 0.5 mg and 25 mg of $MSO_4$ (cumulative). During examination the patient is diaphoretic and anxious. Her BP is 170/100 mm Hg in the right arm and 90/60 mm Hg in the left. Femoral pulses are barely palpable, and her feet are mottled. Chest radiograph reveals a widened mediastinum and a calcified aortic knob. This clinical picture is consistent with:

    a. Cardiac tamponade
    b. Acute pulmonary edema
    c. Pulmonary embolism
    d. Dissecting aortic aneurysm

14. The Duke criteria for diagnosis of endocarditis consists of the assessment of the presence of major and minor criteria. Which of the following combinations is not consistent with definite clinical diagnosis?

    a. Two positive blood cultures with organisms typical of endocarditis and echocardiographic evidence of new regurgitation
    b. Echocardiographic evidence of endocardial involvement, predisposing heart disorder, IV drug abuse and temperature greater than 38°C
    c. History of valvular regurgitation, fever of higher than 38°C, Osler's nodes, Janeway lesions, and serologic evidence of infection consistent with endocarditis
    d. Three positive blood cultures with organisms consistent with endocarditis and a predisposing heart disorder

15. Medical management of dilated cardiomyopathy frequently includes ACE inhibitors, beta adrenergic antagonists, and aldosterone antagonists. The rationale for these drug choices is that they:

    a. Work synergistically to maximize myocardial contractility and output
    b. Block maladaptive compensatory mechanisms that worsen the disease state
    c. Maximize hormonal responses to decreased cardiac output
    d. Inhibit the atrial dysrhythmia likely to result from dilated myocardium

16. In accordance with the current Joint National Committee (JNC) guidelines for the assessment, classification, and management of hypertension, a blood pressure of 150/90 mm Hg is considered a hypertensive urgency if it is associated with:

    a. Microalbuminuria
    b. Acute myocardial infarction

   c.  Medication nonadherence
   d.  Change in mental status

17. S.L. is a 68-year-old male with aortic stenosis. In addition to chest pain, which of the following would indicate an urgent need for aortic valve replacement?

   a.  Aortic calcification
   b.  Left ventricular hypertrophy
   c.  Pulmonary hypertension
   d.  Syncope

18. A 38-year-old female patient presents with history of fatigue and a fever of 10 days duration. Past medical history is negative for heart disease or murmur. The history is noncontributory with the exception of a cosmetic brow lift 6 months ago. Upon physical examination her temperature is 38.8°C, and there is a grade III systolic murmur at the left sternal border. You note subungual hemorrhages and erythematous lesions on the palms and soles. This history and clinical picture is strongly suggestive of:

   a.  Pericarditis
   b.  Endocarditis
   c.  Pericardial effusion
   d.  Pulmonary embolus

19. A 47-year-old male has been admitted for an elective repair of symptomatic hiatal hernia. His past medical history is significant only for hypertension, which has been well controlled with an ACE inhibitor and thiazide diuretic. The ACNP is called to the bedside to evaluate an acute mental status change. Upon examination the patient is confused and lethargic. Assessment reveals no risk factors for delirium—no medications have been administered, there is no sign of infection, and $SaO_2$ on 2 L nasal $O_2$ is 99%. The only abnormal finding is a blood pressure of 162/110 mm Hg. The ACNP knows that management must include:

   a.  Oral clonidine
   b.  A comprehensive metabolic panel

   c.  Intravenous vasodilators
   d.  A 12-lead ECG

20. Who among the following presents the greatest risk factors for development of deep venous thrombosis?

   a.  A 67-year-old male with alcoholic cirrhosis
   b.  An 18-year-old female on combination hormonal contraception
   c.  A 23-year-old paraplegic following motorcycle accident
   d.  A 50-year-old female who smokes almost two packs of cigarettes daily

# ◘ ANSWERS AND RATIONALE

1. **(b)** This clinical and electrocardiographic picture is consistent with atrial fibrillation. In atrial fibrillation the atrial rate is in excess of 350 bpm and is difficult to calculate. The ventricular rate may be low. R to R intervals are irregular. P waves are indistinguishable. The atria are contracting rapidly and are thus unable to refill before ejection. The ventricles are filled inadequately and cardiac output is diminished, producing the symptoms described. There is an irregular ventricular response, and there is a difference between the apical heart rate and the peripheral pulse rate. The absence of p waves rules out atrial flutter, an identifiable rate rules out ventricular fibrillation, and the scenario indicates no ventricular ectopy (Parrillo & Dellinger, 2008).

2. **(c)** In the setting of dysrhythmia, increased perfusion and decreased demand should always be considered, and may be improved via a review of medications and rest/activity balance. Thrombolytic therapy is not indicated in atrial fibrillation, although anticoagulation therapy should be considered and may be indicated in certain circumstances. Decreasing cardiac output and decreasing INR are not appropriate in the setting of atrial fibrillation (Fuster *et al.*, 2006).

3. **(d)** Leads II, III, and aVF all have their positive leads at the foot and are looking up at the inferior aspect of the heart. The anterior wall is represented in the anterior leads (V1 through V6), the posterior in leads I and aVL, and the posterior wall is reflected in right anterior leads (Parrillo & Dellinger, 2008).

4. **(d)** Thrombolytics are not indicated in MI characterized by ST-T wave inversion, also known as subendocardial MI. Age of 72 and absence of confirming enzymes are not contraindications, and BP does not present a contraindication unless it is greater than 180/110 mm Hg (Anderson, 2007; Antman et al., 2008).

5. **(d)** Pericarditis is an inflammatory process that develops in up to 15% of patients 2 to 7 days postacute myocardial infarction. It would be most likely accompanied by a pericardial friction rub. It is not associated with hypoxia. ST elevations in the V leads would suggest anterior wall MI, and a widened mediastinum suggests bleeding into the thorax as with aortic aneurysm (Marino, 2007; McPhee & Papadakis, 2009).

6. **(d)** Concave elevations in the majority of leads is inconsistent with regional ischemia or injury; the addition of a normal physical examination suggests that this presentation is consistent with pericarditis. NSAIDs are the drug of choice to reduce pericardial inflammation. SL NTG is used for acute angina, and beta adrenergic and calcium channel antagonists are both indicated to relieve myocardial work load, which is not an issue in pericarditis (McPhee & Papadakis, 2009).

7. **(c)** This patient exhibits signs and symptoms of acute left CHF. The goals for this patient are to decrease preload to decrease cardiac work, and to improve contractility to optimize heart function. Reducing afterload with ACE inhibitors will be an important part of chronic CHF management, but the immediate priorities in acute failure are to reduce workload by reducing preload and improving function to improve output (Hunt et al., 2005).

8. **(d)** All findings described in "a," "b," and "c" are associated with chronic venous congestion of congestive heart failure, resulting from an insidious increase of pressure from the right heart backward. The diffuse chest wall heaves occur after myocardium in all chambers has hypertrophied to the extent where the force generated by contraction is visible. JVD results from chronically increased pressure in the jugular vein. Redistribution of flow occurs when the pulmonary veins are chronically subjected to high pressure. Abdominal distention and venous hum are consequences of increased pressure in the portal and splanich beds. However, diffuse pulmonary rales and $S_3$ are more often associated with acute pulmonary edema of acute heart failure (Hunt et al., 2005).

9. **(a)** The aortic valve is best auscultated at the second intercostal space, right sternal border. The valve is open during systole, which would produce a stenotic murmur. The pulmonic valve is best auscultated at the second intercostal space, left sternal border, and the mitral and tricuspid valves are auscultated at the fourth and fifth intercostal spaces, respectively (Seidel et al., 2006).

10. **(a)** Cardiac monitors have traditionally and historically been set to monitor lead II because lead II provides the best representation of a normal electrical propagation from right-upper to left-lower portion of the heart. Evidence clearly suggests that the lead should be selected to best visualize the pathology of concern (e.g., $V_1$ for bundle branch blocks); however, actual practice is very

slow to break away from tradition, and lead II is still often used despite the fact that it is not the best view of any given pathology. No lead is any more cost-effective than the other, and the USPS Task Force does not recommend specific leads for monitoring (McPhee & Papadakis, 2009; Parrillo & Denninger, 2008; USPSTS, 2007).

11. **(a)** This clinical picture is clearly consistent with peripheral arterial disease, from the history of arterial disease in the form of CAD and hypertension and the physical findings. In more mild disease (pain that develops after activity), walking to the point of pain followed by rest would be appropriate—but this patient has pain at rest, which is an indication for aggressive angioplasty or revascularization. Anticoagulation would be appropriate for DVT, and compression stockings for chronic venous insufficiency (Fauci, 2007).

12. **(c)** Pulmonary hypertension is a product of strain to the pulmonary vasculature and right heart. Diagnostic assessment reveals indices consistent with right heart strain such as right ventricular dilation, increased hilar/thoracic ratio, and right ventricular hypertrophy. An R/S ratio in $V_1$ is not consistent with right ventricular hypertrophy; in pulmonary hypertension, the R wave would be bigger than the S wave (ratio > 1) in $V_1$ (McPhee & Papadakis, 2009).

13. **(d)** This is a classic dissecting aneurysm. It can be differentiated from an MI or a pulmonary embolism by the chest radiograph findings and the BP discrepancies. Tamponade, pulmonary edema, and pulmonary embolism would not manifest the blood pressure discrepancy, decreased femoral pulses, or mottling. Pulmonary edema would respond to some extent to nitroglycerin and morphine (McPhee & Papadakis, 2009).

14. **(d)** The Duke criteria for definite clinical diagnosis include either (a) two major criteria, (b) one major and three minor criteria, or (c) five minor criteria. Major criteria include two positive blood cultures with organisms typical of endocarditis, three blood cultures with organisms consistent with endocarditis, or echocardiographic evidence. All other criteria included among the answer choices are minor criteria. Choice "d" is the only option that includes only one major and one minor criterion (McPhee & Papadakis, 2009).

15. **(b)** As a function of low cardiac output, sympathetic tone and renin-angiotensin-aldosterone release are upregulated, resulting in vasopressin, aldosterone, and atrial natriuretic peptide. These maladaptive compensatory mechanisms result in fluid retention, which then results in increased vasoconstriction and afterload. Pharmacologic therapy is initiated to block the positive feedback cycle of these maladaptive mechanisms (Hunt, 2005; McPhee & Papadakis, 2009).

16. **(a)** In addition to the stages of hypertension defined by the JNC in accordance with numerical distinction (prehypertension = 120–139 systolic and 80–90 diastolic, stage 1 = 140–159 systolic and 90–99 diastolic, stage 2 $\geq$ 160 systolic or 100 diastolic), the report defines hypertensive urgencies and hypertensive emergencies. A hypertensive urgency is any blood pressure greater than 140/90 accompanied by progressive target organ damage, e.g., renal dysfunction, retinopathy, LVH. A hypertensive emergency is blood pressure greater than 140/90 in the setting of acute target organ damage, e.g., acute MI, dissecting aneurysm, eclampsia, or hypertensive encephalopathy. Medication nonadherence does not define stage or classification (JNC 7, 2004).

17. **(d)** Syncope is an indication of cerebral hypoperfusion. Valve replacement is needed acutely. Aortic calcification is not uncommon in the elderly population, and is not an indication for aggressive surgical intervention. Left ventricular hypertrophy may be a long-term consequence of aortic stenosis, but is not an indication for surgical intervention. Pulmonary hypertension is not associated with aortic valvular disease as it is manifest in right heart consequences (McPhee & Papadakis, 2009).

18. **(b)** This presentation is consistent with endocarditis, which may produce subungual splinter hemorrhages and Janeway lesions—these lesions are painless, erythematous lesions of the palms or soles. Osler nodes (painful, violaceous raised lesions on the fingers, toes, or feet) may also be seen. Fever may be high, or may be lower and sustained. Finally, a new onset murmur, particularly with the associated findings, is clinically suggestive of endocarditis (Cooper, 2007).

19. **(c)** Hypertension and associated encephalopathy is a hypertensive emergency and requires immediate management with intravenous vasodilators, intra-arterial monitoring, and transfer to intensive care. Oral clonidine might be appropriate for hypertensive urgency, but this is an emergency. A comprehensive metabolic panel and 12-lead ECG might be part of the assessment, but they are not management strategies (JNV 7, 2004).

20. **(c)** The primary risk factors for deep vein thrombosis include stasis and polycythemic disorders. The patient with paraplegia presents the greatest risk here. A patient with alcoholic cirrhosis likely has decreased clotting factors and is actually at greater risk for bleeding rather than clotting. While hormonal contraception does present a very slight risk, in an otherwise healthy 18-year-old the risk is minimal. Similarly, a 50-year-old smoker does not have a significantly greater risk than the general population. While a 50-year-old smoker on hormonal contraception would have a higher risk, that is not an option here, and in any event, the paraplegic still has the higher risk (McPhee & Papdakis, 2009).

## ◘ REFERENCES

American College of Chest Physicians (ACCP). (2004). The seventh ACCP conference on antithrombotic and thrombolytic therapy. *Chest, 126,* 163S–696S.

American Heart Association (AHA). (2006). *Advanced cardiovascular life support provider manual.* Dallas, TX: American Heart Association.

Anderson, J. L. *et al.* (2007). ACC/AHA 2007 guidelines for the management of patients with unstable angina and non-ST-segment elevation myocardial infarction: Executive summary. A report of the American College of Cardiology/American Heart Association Task Force on Practice Guidelines (Writing Committee to Revise the 2002 Guidelines for the Management of Patients with Unstable Angina and Non-ST-Segment Elevation Myocardial Infarction). Circulation: *Journal of the American Heart Association, 116,* 803–877.

Antman, E. M. *et al.* (2007). 2007 focused update of the ACC/AHA 2004 guidelines for the management of patients with ST-elevation myocardial infarction: A report of the American College of Cardiology/American Heart Association Task Force on Practice Guidelines (2007 Writing Group to Review New Evidence and Update the 2004 Guidelines for the Management of Patients with ST-Elevation Myocardial Infarction). *Journal of the American College of Cardiology, 51,* 210–247.

Cooper, D. H., Krainik, A. J., Lubner, S. J., & Reno, H. E. L. (2007). *The Washington manual of medical therapeutics* (32nd ed.).

Philadelphia, PA: Lippincott, Williams, & Wilkins.

Fauci, A. S., Braunwald, E., Kasper, D. L., Hauser, S. L., Longo, D. L., Jameson, J. L., & Loscalzo, J. (Eds.). (2008). *Harrison's principles of internal medicine* (17th ed.). New York: McGraw-Hill.

Fraker, T. D. *et al.* (2007). 2007 chronic angina focused update of the ACC/AHA 2002 guidelines for the management of patients with chronic stable angina: A report of the American College of Cardiology/American Heart Association Task Force on Practice Guidelines Writing Group to Develop the Focused Update of the 2002 Guidelines for the Management of Patients with Chronic Stable Angina. *Journal of the American College of Cardiology, 50,* 2264–2274.

Fuster, V. *et al.* (2006). ACC/AHA/ESC 2006 guidelines for the management of patients with atrial fibrillation: A report of the American College of Cardiology/American Heart Association Task Force on Practice Guidelines and the European Society of Cardiology Committee for Practice Guidelines (Writing Committee to Revise the 2001 Guidelines for the Management of Patients with Atrial Fibrillation). *Journal of the American College of Cardiology, 48,* 149–246.

Hunt, S. A. *et al.* (2005). ACC/AHA 2005 guideline update for the diagnosis and management of chronic heart failure in the adult—summary article: A report of the American College of Cardiology/American Heart Association Task Force on Practice Guidelines (Writing Committee to Update the 2001 Guidelines for the Evaluation and Management of Heart Failure). Circulation: *Journal of the American Heart Association, 112,* 1825–1852.

Joint National Committee on Prevention, Detection, Evaluation, and Treatment of High Blood Pressure (JNC). (2004) *7th Report of the JNC.* Washington, DC: National Institutes of Health (update due Summer 2010).

Marino, P. L. (2007). *The ICU book* (3rd ed.). Philadelphia, PA: Lippincott, Williams, & Wilkins.

McPhee, S. J., & Papadakis, M. A. (Eds.). (2009). *Current medical diagnosis and treatment* (48th ed.). New York: McGraw-Hill.

National Cholesterol Education Panel (NCEP). (2002). *Third report of the Expert Panel on Detection, Evaluation, and Treatment of High Blood Cholesterol in Adults (Adult Treatment Panel III).* Washington, DC: National Institutes of Health (update due Summer 2010).

Parrillo, J., & Dellinger, R. (Eds.). (2008). *Critical care medicine: Principles of diagnosis and management in the adult* (3rd ed.). St. Louis: Mosby, Inc.

Seidel, H. M., Ball, J. W., Dains, J. E., & Benedict, G. W. (2006). *Mosby's guide to physical examination* (6th ed.). St Louis: Mosby, Inc.

US Preventive Services Task Force (USPSTF). (2007). *The guide to clinical preventive services: Recommendations of the United States Preventive Services Task Force.* Retrieved on April 5, 2010 from http://www.ahrq.gov/clinic/pocketgd.pdf.

# 7

# Hematologic Disorders

*Ruth M. Kleinpell*

## Select one best answer to the following questions.

1. A 57-year-old male presents with a vague history of fatigue of unknown duration. He has no significant past medical history, and his physical examination is unremarkable. Laboratory assessment reveals an hgb of 10 g/dL and an hct of 29%. The mean corpuscular volume (MCV) is 75 $\mu^3$, and the mean corpuscular hemoglobin concentration (MCHC) is 30%. The ACNP knows that further evaluation of this patient must include:

   a. A serum $B_{12}$ and folate level
   b. A nutrition consult
   c. A complete metabolic panel
   d. Endoscopic evaluation of the upper and lower GI tract

2. A 48-year-old female presents for a complete physical examination; she has not seen a healthcare provider since having gastric bypass surgery 3 years ago. She denies any complaints, and remains happy with her 97 lb weight loss. Thorough evaluation reveals some decreased vibratory sense in the distal extremities. A CBC is significant for an hgb of 10.1 g/dL and hct of 30%. The MCV is 118 $\mu^3$. The ACNP determines that the cause of anemia is probably due to a deficiency of:

   a. Dietary folic acid
   b. Intrinsic factor
   c. Dietary $B_{12}$
   d. Ferritin

3. A 23-year-old female presents to the emergency room with a history of sickle cell anemia. She is in profound pain, and a sickle cell crisis is suspected. Which of the following statements is not accurate with regard to sickle cell crisis?

   a. It frequently presents with shortness of breath and acute pain.
   b. Management measures should include platelet transfusion.
   c. Sickle cell crises can be precipitated by a recent infection.
   d. Narcotic analgesics are often required to relieve crisis pain.

4. The ACNP is performing an admitting history and physical examination of a 66-year-old female being admitted

for evaluation of high fever. The CBC reveals a white blood cell count (WBC) of 45,000 µ³, with 16% neutorophils, 80% lymphocytes, 3% monocytes, 1% eosinophils, and 1% basophils. This presentation is most consistent with:

a. Chronic lymphocytic leukemia
b. Temporal arteritis
c. Urosepsis
d. Acute bacterial endocarditis

5. Which of the following is characteristic of Non-Hodgkin's lymphoma?

a. It is the most common neoplasm seen in patients older than 50 years of age.
b. It can be confirmed with Reed-Sternberg cells in lymph node tissue.
c. It is classified as an acute lymphocytic leukemia.
d. It often presents with painless lymphadenopathy.

6. Kate S., a 28-year-old female, was admitted with a 3-week history of easy bruising and mucosal petechiae. A diagnosis of thrombocytopenia was made after initial laboratory testing revealed a platelet count of 40,000/µL. She reports a sinus infection 1 week ago, after having the flu for 2 weeks. She is currently hypotensive at 90/50 mm Hg, febrile at 101.2°F, and appears septic. Although the results of additional laboratory tests are pending, the probable diagnosis is:

a. Autoimmune thrombocytopenia purpura (ATP)
b. Possible malignant neoplasm
c. Early disseminated intravascular coagulation (DIC)
d. Acute infectious thrombocytopenia

7. Who among the following patients represents the leading cause of cancer morbidity in the US?

a. A 56-year-old male with lung cancer
b. A 72-year-old female with malignant melanoma
c. A 41-year-old female with breast cancer
d. A 48-year-old male with colon cancer

8. Which of the following laboratory assessments is specific for diagnosing sickle cell anemia?

a. The Sickledex test
b. Assessment of peripheral blood smear
c. The CBC differential
d. Hemoglobin electrophoresis

9. A 48-year-old male is admitted to a subacute care facility for aggressive rehabilitation after a motor vehicle accident. He was previously diagnosed with thalassemia. Which of the following is the most likely representation of his hematologic abnormalities?

a. Hgb 9.6 g/dL, MCV 72 µ³, Hgb A$_2$ 6%
b. Hgb 8.4 g/dL, ferritin 42 ng/mL, neutrophils 88%
c. Hgb 10.2 g/dL, MMA level 0.15 µmol/l, and RDW 16%
d. Hgb 7.9 g/dL, Hct 24%, TIBC 200 µg/dL

10. Which of the following statements is accurate with regard to folic acid deficiency anemia?

a. It presents with neurologic symptoms.
b. It results from malabsorption of folic acid.
c. It is a macrocytic, normochromic anemia.
d. It is the most common type of anemia.

## ◻ ANSWERS AND RATIONALE

1. **(d)** This clinical presentation is consistent with iron deficiency anemia, the most common cause of which is slow, chronic blood loss. Given this patient's age, iron deficiency anemia must be further evaluated with endoscopic evaluation of the gut. Folate and B$_{12}$

assessment is not necessary with micro-cytosis, and while a metabolic panel and dietary assessment may be performed, endoscopic evaluation is clearly the most important of the options (McPhee & Papadakis, 2009; Wallach, 2007).

2. **(b)** Pernicious anemia occurs when there is decreased serum $B_{12}$ for red blood cell synthesis. $B_{12}$ is absorbed through the GI mucosa via intrinsic factor produced by parietal cells. In patients with GI surgery, there is a risk of loss of intrinsic cell production, and dietary $B_{12}$ cannot be absorbed. $B_{12}$ is so abundant in virtually all animal products that a dietary deficiency is very unlikely with the exception of vegan patients. Ferritin is a protein synthesized in response to iron stores and is not generally related to macrocytic anemia. Folate deficiency does not produce neurologic symptoms (Fauci, 2007).

3. **(b)** Sickle cell crisis is an acute, periodic exacerbation in which the RBC becomes sickle shaped and causes vessel obstruction. Cellular hypoxia results in tissue ischemia, which causes pain in the extremities, back, chest, abdomen, and joints. Treatment is directed toward the acute and chronic complications of the disease, and includes oxygen for hypoxemia, antibiotics for infection, fluids for dehydration, analgesics for pain, and occasionally RBC transfusions for anemia. Thrombocytosis frequently accompanies sickle cell disease, with platelet counts higher than normal; transfusion of platelets is not indicated (Cooper, 2007).

4. **(a)** This white count and associated lymphocytosis is most consistent with chronic lymphocytic leukemia (CLL). CLL is the most common form of adult leukemia, found most commonly in persons 50 years of age and older. The fever is most likely not related,

and could represent any of the other choices, including sepsis and endocarditis, which are infectious, or temporal arteritis, which is autoimmune and does not produce any WBC elevation. Temporal arteritis is characterized by a high fever, elevated erythrocyte sedimentation rate (ESR), and normal WBC (McPhee & Papadakis, 2009; Wallach, 2007).

5. **(d)** Non-Hodgkin's lymphoma often presents with painless lymphadenopathy, may have a viral etiology, and is the most common neoplasm for persons aged 20 to 40 years. Reed-Sternberg cells are found in Hodgkin's lymphoma. As this name implies, it is a lymphoma, not a leukemia (Cooper, 2007).

6. **(c)** The probable diagnosis given the history, physical findings, and laboratory results is early DIC. DIC varies greatly in clinical severity and may present with either bleeding or thrombosis. Patients presenting with early DIC demonstrate disturbance in hemostasis with easy bruising and petechia on mucosal membranes. Thrombocytopenia (platelets < 150,000/μL), hypofibrinogenemia (fibrinogen < 170 mg/dL), decreased RBC, increased fibrin degradation products (FDP > 45 μg/dL or present at > 1:100 dilution), prolonged PT (> 19 seconds) and PTT (> 42 seconds) are also seen. Although thrombocytopenia is found in ITP, the patient's clinical findings are suggestive of a concurrent infectious process and possible sepsis, conditions that precipitate DIC. Malignant neoplasms do not characteristically present with thrombocytopenia (Marino, 2007).

7. **(c)** The leading cause of cancer morbidity in the US varies according to gender; it is breast in women and prostate in men. Lung cancer is the leading cause of cancer mortality in both genders, but the actual incidence of lung

cancer is lower. More women and men get breast and prostate cancer respectively, but cure rates are much higher, therefore these are the leading causes of morbidity. When lung cancer does occur, it is more often fatal. Colon cancer is the third most common cause of cancer morbidity and mortality. Melanoma does not rank among the first three in terms of morbidity or mortality (USPSTF, 2007).

8. **(d)** Hemoglobin electrophoresis separates the sickled cells and is diagnostic for sickle cell anemia. The Sickledex can identify sickle cell trait/anemia, but does not differentiate between the two. The peripheral smear is diagnostic for some hemolytic anemias, and can suggest sickle cell, but is not diagnostic. The CBC differential is not diagnostic for anemia type (Fauci, 2007; Wallach, 2007).

9. **(a)** Thalessemia is a genetically inherited disorder resulting in abnormal hemoglobin production and hypochromic, microcytic anemia, found in Mediterranean populations. It is characterized by profound microcytosis and elevations of abnormal hgb such as Hgb $A_2$, Hgb F and Hgb H. A ferritin of 42 is actually normal, but a low or low-normal ferritin would suggest iron deficiency anemia. Neutrophilia suggests infection, MMA (methylmalonic acid) ranges between 0.10 and 0.27; elevated levels suggest early pernicious anemia. Elevated RDW (red cell distribution width) suggests a new or evolving anemia, in which new red blood cells are synthesized under different physiologic circumstances than old red blood cells—thalassemia is unchanged from birth. Finally, TIBC is associated with iron abnormalities (McPhee & Papadakis, 2009).

10. **(c)** Folic acid deficiency anemia is a macrocytic, normochromic anemia due to folic acid deficiency, which is caused by inadequate intake or malabsorption of folic acid. Symptoms include fatigue, dyspnea on exertion, pallor, headache, anorexia, and glossitis. Folic acid deficiency anemia is differentiated from pernicious anemia by neurologic symptoms, such as paresthesias and loss of vibratory sense, which are present only in pernicious anemia. It is generally not a problem of malabsorption, but rather a problem of dietary deficiency (Cooper, 2007).

## ◘ REFERENCES

Cooper, D. H., Krainik, A. J., Lubner, S. J., & Reno, H. E. L. (2007). *The Washington manual of medical therapeutics* (32nd ed.). Philadelphia, PA: Lippincott, Williams, & Wilkins.

Fauci, A. S., Braunwald, E., Kasper, D. L., Hauser, S. L., Longo, D. L., Jameson, J. L., & Loscalzo, J. (Eds.). (2008). *Harrison's principles of internal medicine* (17th ed.). New York: McGraw-Hill.

Marino, P. L. (2007). *The ICU book* (3rd ed.). Philadelphia, PA: Lippincott, Williams, & Wilkins.

McPhee, S. J., & Papadakis, M. A. (Eds.). (2009). *Current medical diagnosis and treatment* (48th ed.). New York: McGraw-Hill.

Seidel, H. M., Ball, J. W., Dains, J. E., & Benedict, G. W. (2006). *Mosby's guide to physical examination* (6th ed.). St. Louis: Mosby, Inc.

US Preventive Services Task Force (USPSTF). (2007). *The guide to clinical preventive services: Recommendations of the United States Preventive Services Task Force*. Retrieved on April 5, 2010 from http://www.ahrq.gov/clinic/pocketgd.pdf.

Wallach, J. (2007). *Interpretation of diagnostic tests* (8th ed.). Philadelphia, PA: Lippincott, Williams, & Wilkins.

# 8

# Immunologic Disorders

*Ruth M. Kleinpell*

## Select one best answer to the following questions.

1. A 31-year-old male patient is being discharged after having been treated for *pneumocystis jiroveci pneumoniae*. He reports taking all of his antiretrovirals as ordered, but developed opportunistic infection anyway. Upon admission his $CD4^+$ count was 325 cells/µL and viral load was 2000 copies/mL. Review of his prior records reveals that when he began therapy his viral load was more than 50,000 copies/mL. The ACNP knows that given this information, his medications need to be adjusted due to:

   a. Virologic failure
   b. Immunologic failure
   c. Immune reconstitution syndrome
   d. Intolerance to the current regimen

2. Your patient was diagnosed with HIV. This is his first visit for general health evaluation, counseling, and discussion of treatment. His absolute $CD4^+$ count is 500 cells/µL and viral load is 25,000 copies/mL. With regard to antiretroviral treatment, you tell the patient that based on his laboratory tests:

   a. Antiretroviral treatment is not appropriate at this time.
   b. He should begin a combination of three antiretroviral medications.
   c. He should begin a combination of antiretroviral medications and pneumonia prophylaxis.
   d. He will need genotype and phenotype testing to determine the starting regimen.

3. A 46-year-old female presents to the outpatient clinic complaining of pain in her hands in the mornings. She reports a history of dropping her coffee cup and dropping her toothbrush, and sometimes feels that she just cannot maintain her grip on items. Radiographic assessment reveals bilateral soft tissue swelling of both metacarpals. The ACNP knows that additional assessment findings will likely include:

   a. Rheumatoid factor (RF) +
   b. Antinuclear antibody (ANA) +
   c. Anti-cyclic Citrullinated Peptide Antibodies—anti-(CCP) +
   d. Heberden's nodes +

4. Rheumatoid arthritis (RA) is diagnosed in a 54-year-old female who has a 1-year history of weakness. Which of the following statements is not true regarding rheumatoid arthritis?

   a. Rheumatoid arthritis is a chronic inflammatory disease of the synovial joint and tendon sheath.
   b. Patients with RA have on average an onset of cardiovascular disease 10 years earlier than those without RA.
   c. Morning stiffness and joint pain are characteristic symptoms.
   d. RA results in joint degeneration, which causes deterioration of bone formation at the joint surfaces.

5. Mr. R., a 65-year-old male, presented to the outpatient clinic with a history of a malar discoid rash, photosensitivity, and oral ulcers. The ACNP initiates a screening test for systemic lupus erythematosus, which must include:

   a. Antinuclear antibodies (ANA)
   b. Anti-double stranded (ds) DNA
   c. Extractable nuclear antigens (ENA)
   d. Antiphospholipid antibodies

6. A 13-year-old patient is seen in the emergency department for an acute onset of a generalized rash. The lesions are discrete, raised, and seem to come and go over the patient's trunk and extremities. The rash started 3 days ago. The history is significant only for being treated almost 3 weeks ago with penicillin following a tooth infection. According to the parents the child is not sexually active. The ACNP explains that:

   a. It is important to do a screening test for syphilis because sexual history may be unclear.
   b. The patient will need to be treated with epinephrine and oral prednisone.

   c. Further assessment may reveal a history of pharyngeal erythema irritation and cardiac murmur.
   d. This is consistent with a penicillin allergy and penicillin compounds should be avoided in the future.

7. The ACNP is evaluating a 72-year-old patient in the emergency department who presents with a fever of 102.9°F, erythrocyte sedimentation of rate of 110 mm/hr, white blood cell count (WBC) of 6500 cells/μL, and right-sided jaw pain. The ACNP knows that the next step must include:

   a. Maxillofacial CT scan
   b. Benzathine PCN 1.2 million units IM
   c. Temporal artery biopsy
   d. Prednisone 60 mg po

8. Ms. R., a 21-year-old female, presents with a persistent cough and upper respiratory symptoms for 2 weeks. She has a history of recurrent pneumonia and was treated three times between the ages of 12 and 14, twice as an inpatient. Her medical history is significant for asthma and rhinitis. Which of the following is the least significant aspect of the history when assessing an immunodeficiency?

   a. History of infections
   b. Vaccination history
   c. Family history
   d. Current medications

9. Mr. H. is a 48-year-old male who presents to the emergency room with difficulty breathing. He reports that he experienced a tingling sensation in his lips and began coughing about 1 hour ago, which progressed to wheezing. He has no significant past medical history. His history is significant only for eating at the buffet before symptoms developed. He admits to trying lots of new seafood. The ACNP knows that this is likely an:

a. Asthma attack
b. Anxiety attack
c. Autoimmune reaction
d. Allergic reaction

10. The ACNP is discharging a 25-year-old male patient who was hospitalized for traumatic injuries sustained during a motor vehicle accident, including a splenectomy. The ACNP advises the patient that:

   a. He should not take any vaccinations except those administered by his primary care provider.
   b. Annual influenza vaccination remains safe but antipneumococcal vaccine should be avoided.
   c. Live-virus vaccines will be more effective than inactive vaccines.
   d. He should get annual influenza vaccines.

## ◘ ANSWERS AND RATIONALE

1. **(b)** Because resistance develops so quickly to antiretroviral therapies, the decision to change therapy should be carefully considered. There are certain criteria under which antiretrovirals should be changed. In this instance, the patient demonstrates immunologic failure, in which the CD4+ count remains impaired, and he develops opportunistic infection. Virologic failure is manifest when the patient's viral load rebounds or does not decrease with therapy; that is not the case with this patient. In virologic failure, the viral load is the relevant parameter. Immune reconstitution syndrome is a febrile illness that occurs in some patients following the initiation of antiretroviral therapy—it suggests an improving immune syndrome, and is not an indication to change treatment. Intolerance is manifest as adverse effects that either impair health or impact quality of life to the extent that the patient cannot

tolerate them (CDC, 2007; McPhee & Papadakis, 2009).

2. **(a)** Antiretroviral treatment is indicated in a patient with: (1) a CD4+ count at less than 350 cells/μL regardless of symptoms, (2) AIDS-defining illness or opportunistic infection regardless of CD4+ count, and (3) pregnancy. This patient does not meet these criteria, so no treatment is indicated. In patients for whom therapy is initiated or changed, genotype and phenotype testing are preferred when available. For any patient with a CD4+ count less than 350 cells/μL, prophylactic therapy is also indicated (CDC, 2007).

3. **(c)** This patient has findings consistent with rheumatoid arthritis. The anti-CCP has a higher sensitivity than RF, and is more likely to be positive early in disease. The RF is positive in less than 50% of patients early in disease and less than 85% overall; anti-CCP is positive in up to 40% of patients who are RF–. The ANA is not often positive in RA, and Heberden's nodes are found in patients with osteoarthritis, not rheumatoid arthritis (Bridges, 2006).

4. **(d)** Rheumatoid arthritis is a chronic inflammatory disease of the synovial joint and tendon sheath. The proximal interphalangeal and metacarpophalangeal joints are often affected. Morning stiffness, which lasts several hours, and joint pain or stiffness are common symptoms. RA is a systemic disease that increases risk for a variety of other diseases, and on average the onset of CVC is 10 years earlier. Joint degeneration is consistent with osteoarthritis, not RA (Fauci, 2007; Bridges, 2006).

5. **(a)** Screening for lupus should begin with serum ANA. It is inexpensive and highly sensitive for lupus; more than 90% of patients with lupus will have

it. Because it is not specific to lupus, patients who are ANA positive will need further confirmation testing with anti-dsDNA, which is highly specific— however, due to its expense, it is not a screening tool. ENA tests for many subtypes of autoimmune disease, and is used when diagnosis is unclear. Antiphospholipid antibodies indicate an increased risk of clotting, and may be present in patients with lupus, but is not unique to lupus (McPhee & Papadakis, 2009).

6. **(d)** This is probably a penicillin allergy; rash reactions may occur as long as 3 weeks after the drug is administered. Epinephrine and steroids are not indicated at this point, because respiratory symptoms characteristic of more severe reactions are not delayed by weeks. The patient may need antihistamines depending on severity of symptoms. While it is not appropriate to rely on the parents' knowledge of sexual activity, this rash is not consistent with the rash of secondary syphilis, and syphilis testing is not indicated (Cooper, 2007).

7. **(d)** The patient most likely has temporal arteritis. The triad of fever, high ESR and normal WBC warrants immediate treatment with prednisone in order to reduce the autoimmune inflammation of the temporal artery. Maxillofacial imaging is not indicated. PCN would be useful for some infectious disease, but this is not infectious. A temporal artery biopsy should be requested to confirm diagnosis, but treatment should not be delayed as the optic nerve may infarct, causing permanent blindness. When this clinical triad exists, the patient should begin high dose prednisone immediately, and the biopsy may be obtained within the next week (Cooper, 2007; McPhee & Papadakis, 2009).

8. **(b)** A patient presenting with frequent infections should have a thorough history of all known infections since childhood. Specific pathogens should be documented if known. Family history is an essential factor in diagnosing genetically transmitted disorders. Current medications are also important information as medications such as phenytoin have been known to cause an IgA deficiency that is reversible. Conversely, vaccination history is really not contributory (Cooper, 2007).

9. **(d)** The most likely diagnosis is an allergy attack. The symptoms of tingling sensation, coughing, wheezing, and difficulty breathing indicate an allergic response, possibly related to a food, drink, or smoke allergen. Anxiety attacks may be similar, but there is nothing to indicate an anxiety event at the time of symptom onset, and there are no classic anxiety symptoms, e.g., palpitations. An asthma attack is unlikely given the absence of a medical history. Similarly, there is no evidence of autoimmune disease (Cooper, 2007).

10. **(d)** Asplenia is a risk factor for immunocompromise. Immunocompromised patients, such as those with no spleen, on cancer chemotherapy, with AIDS, or on high-dose steroids, should avoid live virus vaccines (e.g., MMR, BCG). Inactive viruses like influenza vaccine and antipneumococcal vaccine pose no risk and should be highly encouraged. Pneumococcal vaccines will need to be given more frequently when immune responses are impaired (CDC, 1993; USPSTF, 2007).

## ◘ REFERENCES

Bridges, S. L. (2006). Spotting aggressive RA early: The physical examination, testing, and imaging. *Journal of Musculoskelet Medicine, 23* (Suppl Nov), S10–S14.

Centers for Disease Control and Prevention (CDC). (1993). Recommendations of the Advisory Committee on Immunization Practices (ACIP): Use of vaccines and immune globulins in persons with altered immunocompetence. *Morbidity and Mortality Weekly Report.* Retrieved on December, 29, 2009 from http://www.cdc.gov/mmwr/preview/mmwrhtml/00023141.htm.

Centers for Disease Control and Prevention (CDC). (2006). Sexually transmitted diseases treatment guidelines. *Morbidity and Mortality Weekly Report, 55*(No. RR-11), 1–94.

Cooper, D. H., Krainik, A. J., Lubner, S. J., & Reno, H. E. L. (2007). *The Washington manual of medical therapeutics* (32nd ed.). Philadelphia, PA: Lippincott, Williams, & Wilkins.

Fauci, A. S., Braunwald, E., Kasper, D. L., Hauser, S. L., Longo, D. L., Jameson, J. L., & Loscalzo, J. (Eds.). (2008). *Harrison's principles of internal medicine* (17th ed.). New York: McGraw-Hill.

Marino, P. L. (2007). *The ICU book* (3rd ed.). Philadelphia, PA: Lippincott, Williams, & Wilkins.

McPhee, S. J., & Papadakis, M. A. (Eds.). (2009). *Current medical diagnosis and treatment* (48th ed.). New York: McGraw-Hill.

US Preventive Services Task Force (USPSTF). (2007). *The guide to clinical preventive services: Recommendations of the United States Preventive Services Task Force.* Retrieved on April 5, 2010 from http://www.ahrq.gov.clinic/pocketgd.pdf.

# 9

# Endocrine Disorders

*Candis Morrison*

## Select one best answer to the following questions.

1. A 30-year-old patient with a history of type 2 diabetes is brought into the emergency department (ED) in a near comatose state. His heart rate is 124 bpm and BP is 86/50 mm Hg. Initial laboratory evaluation reveals a blood glucose level of 625 mg/dL, with negative serum ketones. Urine glucose is 4+ and ketones are present in the urine. Serum potassium is 4.0 mEq/dL and serum osmolality is 320 mOsm/L. The ACNP knows that immediate treatment must include which of the following?

   a. Humulin R 20 units intravenous push (IVP)
   b. $D_5$1/2 NSS infusion
   c. Humulin R 1 u/kg/hr intravenous drip
   d. Normal saline solution (NSS) infusion

2. A 35-year-old patient with type 1 DM is maintained on a regimen of basal insulin twice daily and premeal ultra-shortacting insulin. Her HgbA1c is

8.1%. A 3-day review of her blood sugar trends is as follows:

| Before Breakfast | Before Dinner |
| --- | --- |
| 109 mg/dL | 210 mg/dL |
| 97 mg/dL | 182 mg/dL |
| 115 mg/dL | 206 mg/dL |

The appropriate intervention would be to:

   a. Increase the predinner ultra-short acting insulin
   b. Increase the prebreakfast long acting insulin
   c. Decrease the prebreakfast ultra-short acting insulin
   d. Decrease the predinner long acting insulin

3. J. M. is a 19-year-old patient who is being managed by the trauma service following a motor vehicle accident that included head impact. There was no obvious head injury, but the patient had a variety of other problems including a puncture wound to the abdomen and a pneumothorax requiring chest tube reexpansion. This morning he developed nausea and increasing

confusion. Physical examination reveals a bounding pulse, tachycardia, and a blood pressure of 140/108 mm Hg. His urine output is only 58 cc for the last four hours. A metabolic panel is significant for a serum $Na^+$ of 121 mEq/L and $K^+$ of 3.2 mEq/L. The ACNP knows that this clinical history and examination are consistent with:

   a. Syndrome of inappropriate antidiuretic hormone (SIADH)
   b. Addisonian crisis
   c. Cushing's syndrome
   d. Myxedema coma

4. Diabetes insipidus (DI) is a condition characterized by a decrease in antidiuretic hormone (ADH). When evaluating the patient with DI, the ACNP might reasonably anticipate:

   a. A urine $Na^+$ of 15 mEq/L and a serum $Na^+$ of 131 mEq/L
   b. A urine osmolality of 1.001 mosm/L and a serum osmolality of 320 mosm/L
   c. Progressive mental status changes resulting in seizure
   d. Progressive tachydysrhythmia resulting in cardiovascular collapse

5. R. J. is a 37-year-old secretary presenting to urgent care with symptoms of severe headache, intermittent palpitations, nausea, vomiting, nervousness, irritability, and dyspnea. Symptoms began abruptly this morning. Her occupational health nurse reports that her BP was 200/110 mm Hg when taken in the clinic before referral. Current medication includes Premarin 0.625 mg q.d. Her status is post-total hysterectomy and bilateral oophorectomy 2 years ago. Past medical history is noncontributory. Objective findings reveal: temperature 37.8°C, BP 160/90 mm Hg sitting and 130/70 mm Hg standing, heart rate 104 bpm sitting and 128 bpm standing, and respiration 24 bpm. Skin is warm and moist. Her chest is clear to auscultation. Cardiovascular examination reveals a regular but rapid rate and a grade II systolic murmur heard best over the precordium. Neurologic examination is unremarkable with the exception of a sustained tremor bilaterally. To differentiate between two possible causes of this symptom complex, which two tests would be most helpful?

   a. Dexamethasone suppression test and an MRI of the brain
   b. Adrenocorticotropic hormone (ACTH) stimulation test and chest CT scan
   c. Glucose tolerance test and erythrocyte sedimentation rate
   d. Thyroid function studies and urinary catecholamines

6. The ACNP is evaluating a patient who has been maintained on long-term oral prednisone therapy for treatment of asthma. The patient reports the development of significant cystic acne, purpose straie, and an increased tendency to bad temper. Which of the following additional findings would the ACNP anticipate?

   a. Increased hair growth and suppressed WBC
   b. Hypertension and hyperglycemia
   c. Weight gain and hyperkalemia
   d. Oligomenorrhea and tachycardia

7. A 49-year-old male complains of intermittent episodes of severe headache and diaphoresis. He reports that his heart often races, and he gets dizzy spells. He has lost 10 pounds over the past 2 to 3 months. Upon examination he demonstrates marked orthostatic hypotension. Ophthalmoscopic examination reveals arterial narrowing. Cardiac auscultation reveals an $S_4$ sound. ECG reveals left ventricular hypertrophy (LVH). Serum multichemical analysis (SMA) 20, thyroid function tests, and CBC with differential are all within normal limits. The ACNP strongly suspects:

   a. Adrenal insufficiency
   b. Renal artery stenosis
   c. Thyroid storm
   d. Pheochromocytoma

8. A 21-year-old male patient presents in the emergency department with very high blood pressure at 220/140 mm Hg. His medical history is negative. Reportedly he was participating in a wrestling match at a local demonstration and was thrown to the mat very hard, landing on his back. He is responsive but confused. He complains of profound headache and heart palpitations. The ACNP orders a(n):

   a. 24-hour urine for metanephrines
   b. Serum catecholamines
   c. Abdominal CT scan
   d. MRI of the head

9. A 33-year-old obese white female returns for her third BP check for a diagnosis of hypertension. On further questioning she complains of polyuria, polyphagia, weight gain, amenorrhea, and easy bruisability. Physical examination reveals truncal obesity, mild hirsutism and bilateral peripheral edema. Laboratory examination reveals a random glucose of 285 mg/dL. The ACNP considers that the most likely diagnosis is:

   a. Diabetes mellitus
   b. Diabetes insipidus
   c. Cushing's disease
   d. Hypothyroidism

10. You are examining a 42-year-old female who claims to have been obese since childhood. She insists that she complies with a prescribed 1500 calorie diet and has tried multiple diets and exercise plans to lose weight. She also complains of cold intolerance, fatigue, constipation, and menorrhagia. Upon physical examination she has coarse, dry skin, her voice is somewhat hoarse, and her deep tendon reflexes demonstrate delayed response. Which test would be the most appropriate to begin her evaluation?

   a. 24-hour urine metanephrines
   b. Thyroid stimulating hormone (TSH)
   c. $T_3$ and $T_4$
   d. Thyroglobulins

11. Your insulin-dependent patient is on split doses of NPH. His morning self-glucose monitoring has consistently revealed elevated morning readings. You order a 3 a.m. glucose, which is also elevated. This implies:

   a. Dawn phenomenon
   b. Smogyi effect
   c. Insulin allergy
   d. Reactive hypoglycemia

12. A 46-year-old woman presents with symptoms of increased sweating, intolerance to heat, increased appetite, and a weight loss of 10 pounds in the preceding 3 weeks. She has been unable to sleep at night and has become irritable. She has missed her last two periods and believes that her symptoms are menopausal. Upon examination her heart rate is rapid at 112 bpm. Her skin is warm and moist. Examination of her neck reveals a diffuse goiter. She has a fine hand tremor. Initial laboratory values reveal a mild normochromic, normocytic anemia, an increased erythrocyte sedimentation rate, and suppressed serum TSH. The ACNP knows that treatment must include:

   a. A Lugol's solution 1 gtt qd
   b. Radioactive ablation of the thryoid gland
   c. Levothyroxine 100 ug/d
   d. Inderal 20 mg q.i.d.

13. A. S. is a 32-year-old patient complaining of headache and diplopia of recent onset. Review of systems reveals a 4-year history of irregular menses and a bilateral milky nipple discharge that is spontaneous. Family history is negative for breast and gynecologic cancers. An important screening test for this patient would be serum:

   a. Prolactin
   b. Metanephrines
   c. Estradiol
   d. Cortisol

14. A male patient presents as stuporous with nonpurposeful responses to assessment. He is hypotensive with a blood pressure of 82/50 mm Hg; pulse is 124 bpm, and the only other remarkable physical finding is a marked absence of axillary and pubic hair. Basic metabolic panel reveals $Na^+$ 124 mEq/dL, $K^+$ 6.3 mEq/dL, Cl of 103 mEq/dL, $CO_2$ of 27 mEq/dL and blood sugar of 64 mg/dL. The ACNP knows that this patient will likely need to be treated with _____ in addition to NSS infusion.

    a.  IV norepinephrine
    b.  IV hydrocortisone
    c.  IV levothyroxine
    d.  IV vasopressin

15. The ACNP has just had a new patient transferred to his service. The patient was originally admitted for management of an adrenocortical crisis. He was treated with glucocorticoid and mineralocorticoid therapy. The ACNP knows that his mineralocorticoid therapy should be titrated down if he develops:

    a.  Palpitations and flushing
    b.  Hypokalemia and neutropenia
    c.  Hypertension and edema
    d.  Hyperpigmentation and hypergonadism

## ◼ ANSWERS AND RATIONALE

1.  **(d)** This patient is experiencing hyperosmolar nonketotic syndrome (HNS). The primary problem is his hyperosmolarity; he is not acidotic as evidenced by the negative serum ketones. Treatment must include an isoosmolar fluid like NSS. D51/2 NSS is not appropriate as the D5 will readily diffuse into interstitium leaving a hypoosmolar solution; while insulin will likely be given to this patient, neither choice offered is appropriate. The 20 units push is too much for any patient, and the IV gtt suggested is for a patient in diabetic ketoacidosis (Cooper, 2007).

2.  **(b)** Insulin replacement therapy in type 1 DM is designed to try and mimic normal physiologic function. This suggests that all patients should maintain a certain basal insulin to ensure normoglycemia, and supplement with premeal short acting insulin to control the postprandial insulin surge. The patient is clearly experiencing hyperglycemia before the evening meal; therefore the prebreakfast long acting dose should be increased, which will prevent the predinner hyperglycemia. If the predinner ultra-short acting is increased, she will remain hyperglycemic before dinner as a long-term trend, increasing her risk of vascular complications (McPhee & Papadakis, 2009).

3.  **(a)** This patient is exhibiting signs and symptoms of free water retention, as evidenced by the hyponatremia, low-normal potassium, bounding pulse, and hypertension. His history of head injury is consistent with inappropriate ADH secretion. This is usually transient and requires supportive management of fluid restriction and occasionally diuresis. Myxedema coma is characterized by some fluid retention but not the characteristic electrolyte abnormality described here. Addison's disease and Cushing's syndrome are disorders of adrenal function not typically preceded by head injury; additionally, the symptom complex of both disorders is rather different (Cooper, 2007; Parrillo & Denninger, 2008).

4.  **(b)** In DI, the problem is that the patient has a deficiency in antidiuretic hormone. Consequently, the kidney cannot conserve water, and the patient loses free water in large volumes. The urine is very wet with low specific gravity, while plasma becomes very dry with high osmolarity. Urine $Na^+$ will be low at less than 5 mEq/L and plasma $Na^+$ will be high at greater than 145 mEq/L (Cooper, 2007).

5.  **(d)** This picture is most consistent with the diagnosis of pheochromocytoma or thyrotoxicosis. With a clinical picture of hypermetabolism, normal thyroid functions ($T_4$, $FT_4$, $T_3$, and TSH) would eliminate the possibility of a thyroid hormone excess, supporting the diagnosis of pheochromocytoma (Cooper, 2007; Fischback & Dunning, 2008).

6.  **(b)** This patient has iatrogenic Cushing's syndrome as a result of the prednisone therapy. The metabolic effects of cortisol include increased vascular tone, mobilization of glucose, increased free water clearance, and suppression of inflammation. Consequently, expected findings in excess include hyperglycemia, hypokalemia, hypertension, and leukocytosis (Guyton, 2006; McPhee & Papadakis, 2009).

7.  **(d)** These signs and symptoms are consistent with pheochromocytoma. The manifestations of pheochromocytoma are varied. It typically causes attacks with severe headache, palpitations, tachycardia, profuse sweating, vasomotor changes, precordial or abdominal pain, increasing nervousness and irritability, increased appetite, and loss of weight. Physical findings may include hypertension, either in attacks or sustained, and often severe. Patients may show cardiac enlargement, postural tachycardia and hypotension. Adrenal insufficiency presents as hypotension, renal artery stenosis as hypertension without the other symptoms, and thyroid storm manifests with a variety of noncardiogenic excesses, such as extreme weight loss, oligomenorrhea, tremor, and confusion (Cooper, 2007; Fauci, 2007; Guyton, 2006).

8.  **(c)** This clinical presentation is consistent with pheochromocytoma, a catecholamine-producing tumor of the adrenal medulla. Given the acuity of the situation, an abdominal CT should be done to look for the tumor. If the patient were being assessed as a stable outpatient, a 24-hour urine for urinary metabolites would be indicated. Serum catecholamines are metabolized very quickly and are not a reliable indicator of disease (Parrillo & Denninger, 2008).

9.  **(c)** Cushing's disease presents with symptoms of amenorrhea, polydipsia, polyuria, and signs of hypertension, acne, central obesity, and impaired glucose tolerance. Diabetes mellitus presents as hyperglycemia and associated vascular consequences, diabetes insipidus is a condition characterized by profound volume loss and associated symptoms of dehydration, and hypothyroid presents as weight gain, cold intolerance, low pulse, blood pressure, and a general picture of hypometabolism (McPhee & Papadakis, 2009).

10. **(b)** This clinical picture is consistent with hypothyroidism. The TSH is considered the most sensitive indicator of thyroid function, will be increased in primary hypothyroidism, and is the appropriate screening test. Metanephrines are used to screen for pheochromocytoma, and thyroglobulins, as well as $T_3$ and $T_4$, are subsequent tests that may be ordered later to differentiate among specific causes of thyroid disease (Fischbach & Dunning, 2008; McPhee & Papadakis, 2009).

11. **(a)** To differentiate between the dawn phenomenon and the Smogyi effect (two causes of a.m. hyperglycemia) a 3 a.m. glucose is ordered. When it is high, this implies nocturnal insensitivity to insulin, known as the dawn phenomenon. Effective management includes an increase in the p.m. basal insulin. If the 3 a.m. glucose is low, that would suggest that a nocturnal hypoglycemia was occurring and that counterregulatory release of glucagon, cortisol, and epinephrine subsequently raised sugar to higher than necessary levels. This is known as the Smogyi effect, and

treatment is to decrease the p.m. basal insulin so that nocturnal hypoglycemia will not occur (McPhee & Papadakis, 2009).

12. **(d)** This patient has symptomatic hyperthyroidism and must be treated with a noncardioselective beta adrenergic antagonist for symptom control. Depending upon identified cause, she may be treated with radioactive ablation or surgery. Lugol's solution is a temporary measure to decrease the vascularity of the gland preoperatively. Levothyroxine is indicated for hypothyroidism (Fauci, 2007).

13. **(a)** The major concern in this case is a prolactin secreting macroadenoma known as prolactinoma. If this were the cause of the symptoms, serum prolactin would be elevated in excess of 250 ng/mL. This should prompt MRI evaluation and neurosurgical referral. Metanephrines would be the screening for a pheochromocytoma, which would not result in nipple discharge. Similarly, cortisol would screen for Cushing's syndrome, which would not produce nipple discharge. Abnormalities of estrogen could contribute to abnormal menses and failure to conceive, but would not produce nipple discharge (Cooper, 2007; McPhee & Papadakis, 2009).

14. **(b)** The hyponatremia, hyperkalemia, hypotension, and lack of response to isotonic saline infusion are all strongly consistent with an Addisonian crisis, or acute deficiency of adrenalcortical hormone. The patient will need an IV infusion of hydrocortisone in order to restore vascular tone and the ability to retain fluid. The patient will not respond to vasopressors. Levothyroxine will be appropriate in a hypothyroid crisis, and vasopressin may be indicated in diabetes insipidus (Parrillo & Denninger, 2008).

15. **(c)** The mineralocorticoid that is replaced is fludrocortisone, which is a powerful hormone of salt retention. It is dosed very minimally, begun at 0.05 mg three times weekly, and titrated up slowly. If the patient develops clinical signs of acute fluid overload, the drug should be titrated down and/or discontinued. It is not typically required for chronic management, and is frequently added to the chronic cortisol replacement in episodes of acute crisis (Parrillo & Denninger, 2008).

# ◘ REFERENCES

Cooper, D. H., Krainik, A. J., Lubner, S. J., & Reno, H. E. L. (2007). *The Washington manual of medical therapeutics* (32nd ed.). Philadelphia, PA: Lippincott, Williams, & Wilkins.

Fauci, A. S., Braunwald, E., Kasper, D. L., Hauser, S. L., Longo, D. L., Jameson, J. L., & Loscalzo, J. (Eds.). (2008). *Harrison's principles of internal medicine* (17th ed.). New York: McGraw-Hill.

Fischbach, F., & Dunning, M. B. (2008). *A manual of laboratory and diagnostic tests* (8th ed.). Philadelphia, PA: Lippincott, Williams, & Wilkins.

Guyton, A. C., & Hall, J. E. (2006). *Textbook of medical physiology* (11th ed.). Philadelphia, PA: Saunders.

Marino, P. L. (2007). *The ICU book* (3rd ed.). Philadelphia, PA: Lippincott, Williams, & Wilkins.

McPhee, S. J., & Papadakis, M. A. (Eds.). (2009). *Current medical diagnosis and treatment* (48th ed.). New York: McGraw-Hill.

Parrillo, J., & Dellinger, R. (Eds.). (2008). *Critical care medicine: Principles of diagnosis and management in the adult* (3rd ed.). St. Louis: Mosby, Inc.

# 10

# Gastrointestinal Disorders

*Ruth M. Kleinpell*

## Select one best answer to the following questions.

1. Ms. R., a 47-year-old female, presents with a 4-week history of dyspepsia. She denies abdominal pain, but admits to an uncomfortable, gnawing sensation that worsens when she eats. She has tried over the counter (OTC) antacids with limited success. She has no significant medical history. Which feature of her history indicates that an endoscopy should be performed?

   a. Age
   b. Gender
   c. Symptoms worse after eating
   d. Limited response to OTC drugs

2. A 47-year-old female presents complaining of nausea and vomiting with discomfort in her right-upper quadrant and scapular region. Further evaluation reveals that she has had these episodes before, and thinks she was told that she had cholecystitis, but she never followed up on it. The ACNP expects which of the following additional findings?

   a. A + HIDA scan
   b. A – Murphy's sign
   c. A palpable gallbladder
   d. Jaundice

3. A 76-year-old male is being evaluated for profound abdominal pain. His history is significant for coronary artery disease with myocardial infarction at age 68. He continues to smoke one pack per day, and is currently managed for his heart disease with metoprolol. He was in his usual state of health until this a.m. when he developed severe, generalized, abdominal pain. The abdominal exam is unremarkable, but his blood pressure is 88/58 and pulse is 110 bpm. The stool is heme positive. The ACNP suspects:

   a. Ruptured appendix
   b. Perforated ulcer
   c. Mesenteric ischemia
   d. Peritonitis

4. Mr. J. is a 32-year-old male who presents with a 4-day history of fever, left-lower abdominal pain and tenderness, and diarrhea. He denies any

history of colon problems. The most likely diagnosis is:

a. Crohn's disease
b. Diverticulitis
c. Ulcerative colitis
d. Ischemic colitis

5. G.Y. is a 22-year-old male patient who comes to the emergency room for the second time in a 24-hour period. He came in yesterday complaining of abdominal discomfort, but his exam was essentially benign, and routine laboratory screening was within normal limits. Today he reports the pain has "moved" to an area that he indicates in the right-lower quadrant. His white blood cell count is 16,000 cells/μL, and his temperature is 101.3°F. Physical examination reveals pain when the right hip and knee are flexed and the right hip is rotated internally. This physical finding is known as:

a. McBurney's sign
b. The obturator sign
c. The psoas sign
d. Murphy's sign

6. Peritonitis is suspected in a 66-year-old female in the emergency room. Which of the following findings is not an abdominal manifestation of peritonitis?

a. Pain
b. Distention
c. Rigidity
d. Rebound pain

7. A 45-year-old female patient is being evaluated in the emergency department. She presents as just "overall sick" and upon evaluation is found to have a history significant for profound alcohol abuse. Her mental status appears to be deteriorating, and acute liver failure is suspected. The ACNP knows that which of the following criteria will confirm acute liver failure?

a. + HIDA scan, PT > 60 seconds, and age > 40
b. PT > 50 seconds, jaundice of > 1 week duration, and bilirubin > 17.5 mg/dL

c. AST to ALT ratio > 1, bilirubin > 15 mg/dL, and + ultrasound
d. ALT > 10,000 u, PT > 15 seconds, esophageal varices

8. A 27-year-old male presents complaining of fatigue and profound nausea. The physical exam is significant only for mild, nonspecific upper-abdominal discomfort to palpation. The ACNP perceives a faint discoloration to the sclera but is uncertain as to whether it is a normal variant or early jaundice. Laboratory assessment reveals significantly elevated transaminases. A hepatitis profile is as follows:

+ anti-HAV IgM
+ HBsAg
+ anti-HBcAg
+ anti-HBeAg
+HCV RNA
+ anti-HCV

The ACNP expects that the history will be significant for:

a. Travel to Mexico within the last 6 weeks
b. Unprotected sex with a new partner in the last 4 weeks
c. Intravenous drug use within the last 6 months
d. Eating at a seafood buffet within the last 4 months

9. The ACNP is examining a patient who was initially admitted for GI bleeding due to peptic ulcer disease. Bleeding resolved with conservative intervention 2 days ago, and the patient is prepared for discharge today. However, this a.m. the patient is found to be febrile, and although she does not have significant abdominal pain, she has a distended, rigid abdomen with rebound tenderness to palpation. Further diagnostic evaluation should *not* include:

a. Abdominal ultrasound
b. CBC with white blood cell differential
c. CT scan of the abdomen
d. A barium swallow

10. A 54-year-old female is being evaluated for acute abdominal pain. She reports that she has felt unwell for the last day or two, that the pain is steady and seems to travel to her back. Laboratory assessment reveals an amylase of greater than three times the upper limit of normal (ULN) and lipase greater than five times ULN. Abdominal radiograph reveals a gas-filled duodenum. Upon physical exam the ACNP may expect to discover which of the following?

a. Murphy's sign
b. Psoas sign
c. Cullen's sign
d. McBurney's sign

11. A 42-year-old male presents to the clinic with bloody diarrhea. He admits to chronic lower abdominal discomfort, and history reveals a 5 lb weight loss over the previous year. Examination of the rectum demonstrates some excoriation. The ACNP knows that the best diagnostic study to confirm the diagnosis would be:

a. CT scan
b. Barium enema
c. HIDA scan
d. Colonoscopy

12. Bowel obstruction can vary in its presentation depending upon the patient's general state of health, location of the obstruction, and time since onset. Which of the following physical findings is not seen in any typical bowel obstruction scenario?

a. Cramping abdominal pain
b. Abdominal distention
c. High-pitched, tinkling bowel sounds
d. Rebound tenderness

13. Assessment of abdominal pain can be a significant clinical challenge requiring careful assessment of contributory information. The ACNP knows that which of the following associated findings is consistent with a surgical abdomen?

a. Vomiting precedes the onset of pain.
b. Vomiting does not occur.
c. Vomiting occurs after the pain onset.
d. Vomiting is a prominent feature.

14. Mr. S., a 49-year-old male, is brought to the emergency room by his roommate, who relates that the patient has been vomiting bright red blood for 2 days. He has a history of alcohol abuse. Current vital signs are as follows: temperature 99.2°F, heart rate 110 bpm (sinus tachycardia), blood pressure 90/60 mm Hg, respiration 32 bpm. He is alert but lethargic and denies current abdominal pain. Which of the following is not indicated in the initial management of this patient?

a. Immediate IV access
b. Laboratory screening, type and cross-match
c. Endoscopy
d. Crystalloid infusion

15. The ACNP is performing an initial history and physical examination on a 29-year-old female who is new to the practice. She is 5 ft 5 in and 160 lbs, which the ACNP knows is more than 20% above ideal body weight. Which of the following represents the next best action?

a. Discuss with the patient the need for a nutrition consult
b. Explore the patient's perception of her weight and its health implications
c. Consider screening laboratory assessment for thyroid disease
d. No action is required relative to her weight as her BMI is less than 30

16. Which of the following statements is true with respect to stress ulcer prophylaxis?

a. All patients hospitalized for more than 5 days should have pharmacologic prophylaxis of stress ulcers.

b. Stress ulcer prophylaxis should be given to any hospitalized patient on more than 100 mg of hydrocortisone or equivalent per day.

c. All patients on mechanical ventilation should have pharmacologic stress ulcer prophylaxis.

d. There is no level I evidence that pharmacologic stress ulcer prophylaxis improves outcomes in any patient population.

17. Esophageal varices is a common etiology of upper gastrointestinal bleeding, and may develop due to a wide variety of hepatic and prehepatic causes. Which of the following is the treatment of choice for esophageal varices discovered before gastrointestinal bleeding has occurred?

a. Sclerotherapy or banding

b. Vasopressin

c. Balloon tamponade for controlled bleeding

d. Noncardioselective beta blockade

18. R. M. is a 51-year-old male patient with a long history of progressive liver disease as a consequence of chronic hepatitis infection and alcoholism. He has decompensated significantly in the last few months, and now presents with a variety of vague, general, systemic symptoms including fatigue, nausea, and agitation. Physical examination reveals asterixis, ascites, and fetor hepaticus. The ACNP expects that laboratory assessment will reveal:

a. Normal alkaline phosphatase, normal GGT, prolonged PT

b. AST/ALTs > 5 x ULN, elevated bilirubin, and elevated alkaline phosphatase

c. Hyperbilirubinemia, microcytic anemia, and hypoalbuminemia

d. Increased albumin, increased GGT, increased AST/ALT

19. According to the USPS Task Force and American Cancer Society recommendations, the ACNP knows that screening for colon cancer should:

a. Include colonoscopy

b. Begin at age 50

c. Include sigmoidoscopy when there is bright red bleeding per rectum

d. Be deferred during treatment for peptic ulcer disease

20. Mrs. R. was admitted to the general medical service last week for intravenous antibiotic management of an infected diabetic ulcer. Today she has developed frequent, watery diarrhea. The ACNP orders a stool specimen for:

a. Ova and parasites

b. Occult blood

c. *Clostridium difficile*

d. *Escherichia coli*

## ◘ ANSWERS AND RATIONALE

1. **(c)** This patient has symptoms consistent with peptic ulcer disease (PUD). Typical ulcers—e.g., duodenal ulcers—do not require immediate endoscopic evaluation; a treatment regimen based upon clinical assessment is appropriate. However, if the presentation suggests gastric ulcers, an endoscopy should be performed as the risk of malignancy is higher with gastric ulcers. Presenting features that suggest gastric vs duodenal ulcer include age older than 55 years, symptoms unresponsive to prescribed treatment, or symptoms that exacerbate with eating. Classic duodenal ulcer presentation includes age between 30 and 55 years, good response to prescribed treatment, and symptoms typically improving with ingestion of food or liquid (McPhee & Papadakis, 2009).

2. **(a)** This scenario is consistent with cholecystitis, which occurs most commonly in middle-aged women of Western European descent who are

overweight. The ACNP would expect a + Murphy's sign, which is pain and a sharp intake of breath with right-upper quadrant palpation. It is not typical to palpate the gallbladder, and while jaundice may occur, it is not expected. Initial imaging is with ultrasound, which is positive in approximately 80% of cases. The HIDA scan is a more specific test, used when the ultrasound and clinical examination are inconsistent. In cholecystitis, the HIDA scan will be positive (Cooper, 2007; Seidel *et al.*, 2006).

3. **(c)** The profound abdominal pain, history of arterial disease, heme + stool, hypotension, and pain disproportionate to findings should provoke a leading differential of mesenteric ischemia. This requires immediate surgical intervention. Ruptured appendix and perforated ulcer would both produce typical findings of a surgical abdomen, as well as fever. Peritonitis would not produce this profound pain and hypotension (Parrillo & Denninger, 2008).

4. **(b)** Diverticulitis is characterized by fever and left-lower abdominal pain. While the other answer choices shown also frequently cause lower abdominal discomfort and may produce a low grade temperature, they are also typically characterized by blood in stool and more generalized lower abdominal pain. While diverticulitis may produce blood in stool, this only occurs in approximately 25% of cases. The fact that this patient's pain is confined to the left-lower quadrant and the absence of blood in presentation makes "b" the best answer choice (McPhee & Papadakis, 2009).

5. **(b)** The obturator sign is pain with flexion of the right knee and hip and with internal rotation of the hip. It is indicative of appendicitis. The psoas sign is pain with flexion of the right hip and knee without the internal

rotation. McBurney's sign is right-lower abdominal pain one-third the distance from the iliac crest to the umbilicus and is also characteristic of appendicitis. Murphy's sign is appreciated with right-upper quadrant palpation and suggests cholecystitis (Fauci, 2007; Seidel *et al.*, 2006).

6. **(d)** Clinical manifestations of peritonitis include abdominal pain, distention, and rigidity. Anorexia, nausea and vomiting, fever, and chills can also be present. However, rebound tenderness is the hallmark finding of a surgical abdomen, and is not present in peritonitis (Cooper, 2007).

7. **(b)** Acute liver failure is generally rapidly developing and can occur as a function of acetaminophen overdose or nonacetaminophen overdose. Predictors of acute liver failure are as follows: a PT of greater than 100 seconds, and any three of the following five criteria are independent predictors: (1) age younger than 10 years or older than 40 years; (2) fulminant hepatic failure due to non-A, non-B, non-C hepatitis; halothane hepatitis; or idiosyncratic drug reactions; (3) jaundice present longer than 1 week before onset of encephalopathy; (4) PT greater than 50 seconds; and (5) serum bilirubin greater than 300 mmol/L (17.5 mg/dL) (Sood, 2009; Wallach, 2007).

8. **(a)** This patient's laboratory panel reveals acute infection with hepatitis A and chronic infection with hepatitis B and C; therefore, symptoms are most likely a result of the acute infection. Hepatitis A is an enteral hepatitis, commonly linked to shellfish or travel to Mexico or other endemic countries. The incubation period is 2 to 6 weeks—therefore the ACNP expects that exposure to enteral hepatitis has occurred within the last 2 to 6 weeks. Parenteral hepatitis infection, such as B and C, have incubation periods of 6 weeks to

6 months. The potential sexual exposure 4 weeks ago is too soon to produce symptoms, and while IV drug use 4 months ago could cause infection with hepatitis B or C, the acute symptoms are more likely due to the hepatitis A, making "a" the best answer of those provided (McPhee & Papadakis, 2009).

9. **(d)** The CT scan is the best way to diagnose perforated ulcer, but an ultrasound is not contraindicated. The WBC count elevates very quickly and is a useful marker for impending sepsis. The test that is contraindicated is a barium swallow, as it is not appropriate to introduce barium into a bowel that is communicating with the peritoneum (Cooper, 2007).

10. **(c)** This clinical scenario is suggestive of acute pancreatitis. Upon physical examination the ACNP may appreciate Cullen's sign, which is bluish-discoloration in the area of the umbilicus and indicates some retroperitoneal bleeding. Murphy's sign is suggestive of cholecystitis and is characterized by pain and a sharp intake of breath with right-upper quadrant palpation. McBurney's sign is pain/rebound tenderness with right-lower quandrant palpation suggestive of appendicitis, and the psoas sign is abdominal pain with flexion of the right hip and knee, also suggestive of appendicitis (Cooper, 2007; Seidel *et al.*, 2006).

11. **(d)** This presentation is consistent with ulcerative colitis. Diagnostic examination includes colonoscopy with direct visualization of transmural ulceration of the colon wall. Barium enema and CT scan would be supportive, but are not the best choice of those provided. A HIDA scan is technetium imaging of the gallbladder and would not aid in evaluation of these symptoms (McPhee & Papadakis, 2009).

12. **(d)** Physical findings in bowel obstruction include cramping abdominal pain, abdominal distention, and high pitched, tinkling bowel sounds. Rebound tenderness is a classic finding of a surgical abdomen, and is not necessarily present in obstructed bowel. Many causes of bowel obstruction are not surgical, such as adhesions, ileus, and pseudoobstruction (Fauci, 2007; McPhee & Papadakis, 2009; Parrillo & Denninger, 2008).

13. **(c)** Among all of the associated signs and symptoms that should be assessed, it is important to know whether or not vomiting has occurred, the extent to which it has occurred, and its timing in relationship to the pain. In the case of most surgical abdomens, vomiting is not a prominent feature, and when it occurs it is hours after the onset of pain. When vomiting precedes pain or occurs at the onset of pain, a surgical problem is much less likely (Cooper, 2007).

14. **(c)** Initial steps in management of GI bleeding include obtaining IV access, laboratory screening, and type and cross-match. Patients with hemodynamic compromise should be given immediate volume replacement. Endoscopy would not be an initial assessment but would be indicated for continued bleeding. Otherwise, it is performed after the patient is stabilized and bleeding has stopped (Marino, 2007; Parrillo & Denninger, 2008).

15. **(b)** According to the American Academy of Family Physicians, as with all prevention, obesity counseling should begin early. The recommendation is to begin when the patient is greater than or equal to 20% over ideal body weight. It is most appropriate to begin with an exploration of the patient's perception of her weight and its implications, as that will guide any further assessment and intervention (McInnis *et al.*, 2003).

16. **(c)** According to AHRQ guidelines, stress ulcer prophylaxis should be instituted for all patients with (1) mechanical ventilation, (2) coagulopathy, (3) traumatic brain injury, or (4) major burn injury (level 1). It should also be instituted for all ICU patients with (1) multisystem trauma, (2) sepsis, or (3) acute renal failure (level 2), or (4) an injury severity score (ISS) of more than 15, or (5) patients on more than 250 mg hydrocortisone or equivalent daily (Guillamondegui et al., 2008).

17. **(d)** Options a, b, and c are all reasonable initial interventions for bleeding esophageal varices. However, if diagnosed before bleeding occurs, the use of noncardioselective beta blockade can reduce the risk of bleeding by up to 45%. Dose is determined by a decrease in resting heart rate of 25%, decrease of heart rate to 55 bpm, or development of adverse effects (Cooper, 2007).

18. **(a)** By the time that hepatic cells degenerate into cirrhosis, they are unable to produce some of the markers suggestive of acute disease. The transaminases (ALT/AST) are either normal or just modestly elevated. The GGT and alkaline phosphatase are also frequently normal. Common markers of end-stage cirrhosis include prolonged PT, low albumin, and when anemia occurs, it is normocytic (Schaffer, 2007).

19. **(b)** Both of these organizations recommend screening beginning at age 50. Recommendations on colonoscopy as a screening tool vary, and it is not universally recommended as a routine screening measure. Sigmoidoscopy is useful for the evaluation of symptomatic bright red bleeding per rectum, but does not improve detection with stool guaiac and should not be used alone. Screening should not be deferred for patients being treated for peptic ulcer disease (USPSTF, 2007).

20. **(c)** *Clostridium difficile* diarrhea can occur after beginning antibiotic therapy, usually 4 to 9 days after initiation, but symptoms can occur up to 6 weeks after antibiotics are discontinued. Given the recent antibiotic management, this is the most likely diagnosis. Ova and parasites are much less common, and stool for occult blood is not indicated in initial workup. When watery diarrhea occurs as a consequence of *E. coli*, there are usually other classic symptoms and a rapidly progressive course (Marino, 2007).

◻ **REFERENCES**

Cooper, D. H., Krainik, A. J., Lubner, S. J., & Reno, H. E. L. (2007). *The Washington manual of medical therapeutic*s (32nd ed.). Philadelphia, PA: Lippincott, Williams, & Wilkins.

Fauci, A. S., Braunwald, E., Kasper, D. L., Hauser, S. L., Longo, D. L., Jameson, J. L., & Loscalzo, J. (Eds.). (2008). *Harrison's principles of internal medicine* (17th ed.). New York: McGraw-Hill.

Guillamondegui, O. D., Gunter, O. L., Bonadies, J. A., Coates, J. E., Kurek, S. J., De Moya, M. A., Sing, R. F., & Sori, A. J. (2008). *Practice management guidelines for stress ulcer prophylaxis.* Chicago: Eastern Association for the Surgery of Trauma (EAST).

Marino, P. L. (2007). *The ICU book* (3rd ed.). Philadelphia, PA: Lippincott, Williams, & Wilkins.

McInnis, K. J., Franklin, B. A., & Rippe, J. M. (2003). Counseling for physical activity in overweight and obese patients. *American Family Physician, 67,* 1249–1256, 1266–1268.

McPhee, S. J., & Papadakis, M. A. (Eds.). (2009). *Current medical diagnosis and treatment* (48th ed.). New York: McGraw-Hill.

Parrillo, J., & Dellinger, R. (Eds.). (2008). *Critical care medicine: Principles of diagnosis and management in the adult* (3rd ed.). St. Louis: Mosby, Inc.

Schaffer, E. A. (2007). Cirrhosis. *The Merck Manual.* Retrieved on November 30, 2009 from F:\Zip Drive Backup 4.16.05\Jones & Bartlett\ACNP Book\Cirrhosis Fibrosis and Cirrhosis Merck Manual Professional.mht.

Seidel, H. M., Ball, J. W., Dains, J. E., & Benedict, G. W. (2006). *Mosby's guide to physical examination* (6th ed.). St. Louis: Mosby, Inc.

Sood, G. K. (2009). Acute liver failure. *Emedicine.* Retrieved on December 12, 2009 from http://emedicine.medscape.com/article/177354-overview.

US Preventive Services Task Force (USPSTF). (2007). *The guide to clinical preventive services: Recommendations of the United States Preventive Services Task Force.* Retrieved on April 5, 2010 from http://www.ahrq.gov.clinic/pocketgd.pdf.

Wallach, J. (2007). *Interpretation of diagnostic tests* (8th ed.). Philadelphia, PA: Lippincott, Williams, & Wilkins.

# 11

# Renal/Genitourinary Disorders, STDs

*Ruth M. Kleinpell*

## Select one best answer to the following questions.

1. Mary P., an 18-year-old female, presents to the ED with a 3-day history of dysuria and low back pain. She denies any previous episodes. A urinalysis reveals greater than 3⁺ leukocytes. Urine leukocyte esterase and nitrites are positive. She is currently febrile at 101.8°F and reports having chills last evening. The most likely diagnosis is:

   a. Cystitis
   b. Gonorrhea
   c. Pyelonephritis
   d. Bacterial vaginosis

2. A patient is found to have an asymptomatic rash on both upper extremities. He denies any high-risk sexual activity, but because of the character of the rash, the ACNP asks the patient to be tested for syphilis. He agrees, and a venereal disease research laboratory (VDRL) screening test is performed and found to be positive. Subsequent confirmation testing with the fluorescent treponemal antigen-antibody (FTA-Abs)

test is negative. The patient is advised that:

   a. He is infected but not infectious to others.
   b. He will require repeat testing.
   c. He does have syphilis.
   d. He does not have syphilis.

3. The ACNP is called to see a patient on an inpatient stepdown unit for oliguria. The patient underwent a transurethral resection of the prostate (TURP) 2 days ago. The nurse reports that the urine was straw colored without clots during the previous shift. There is no return from a 100 cc sterile foley irrigation. The patient is alert and reports no discomfort. The operative report indicates the patient had an episode of intraoperative hypotension but vital signs have been stable since. How would the ACNP best differentiate prerenal vs intrarenal oliguria?

   a. Administer a fluid bolus of 500 cc 0.9% NSS and monitor the response
   b. Order an additional 100 cc sterile foley irrigation

c.  Obtain a renal ultrasound

d.  Obtain urine sodium and (fractional excretion of sodium) $FE_{Na+}$ determination

4.  A 45-year-old male presents to the outpatient clinic for a pre-employment physical examination. Laboratory findings are suggestive of stage 2 chronic kidney disease (CKD). The ACNP knows that stage 2 CKD:

a.  Represents 50% nephron loss

b.  Is usually asymptomatic

c.  Is reversible with early detection and treatment

d.  Results in a compensatory increase in glomerular filtration rate (GFR)

5.  Renal failure occurs when there is a decrease in renal function with a resultant retention of urea nitrogen and creatinine in the blood. A variety of physiologic insults can cause this decrease in function, and are classified as one of three types: prerenal, intrarenal, and postrenal. Differentiating the type is necessary to identify appropriate treatment. Which of the following is characteristic of postrenal failure?

a.  It can be reversed when the underlying cause of hypoperfusion is corrected.

b.  It damages the epithelial basement membrane, which can regenerate.

c.  It progresses to intrarenal failure in several days.

d.  It occurs due to mechanical or functional urine flow obstruction.

6.  Knowledge of sexually transmitted infection (STI) is important for the ACNP regardless of practice site as STI represents a significant health condition for millions of Americans. The most common sexually transmitted disease in the US is:

a.  Gonorrhea

b.  Herpes

c.  Human papilloma virus (HPV)

d.  Chlamydia

7.  A 32-year-old male presents complaining of penile discharge and dysuria. He is very concerned because last weekend he attended a bachelor party and was unfaithful to his wife for the first and only time and did not use protection. Upon physical examination the ACNP appreciates copious purulent discharge. A culture is sent to the laboratory; however, given the history and clinical findings, the ACNP counsels the patient that he must tell his wife immediately because he likely has a condition that:

a.  Is the leading cause of infertility in US females

b.  Will require 14 to 28 days of antibiotic treatment

c.  Frequently produces profound symptoms in women

d.  Requires treatment of all contacts

8.  The ACNP is counseling a couple following diagnosis of primary herpes simplex (HSV) 2 virus in the male partner. They are both very upset, because they are both adamant that they have been monogamous for over 2 years, and neither partner has ever had HSV-2 before. Serology reveals that the male partner is HSV-2 IgM positive and the female is HSV-2 IgG positive. This couple should be advised that:

a.  There is no evidence that anyone has been unfaithful; it appears that the female partner had the infection first and infected the male—she may have been infected years ago and not been aware.

b.  They both need to be treated with a course of antiviral agents as IgM represents acute infection, and they may actually pass it back and forth if not treated.

c.  The male partner is only recently infected, and the virus can be eradicated with prompt antiviral treatment; the female has chronic infection for which antiviral therapy is not effective.

d.  They may want to consider couples counseling as it appears that there may be some issues that need to be resolved.

9.  R. M. is a 41-year-old male patient being managed by the ACNP for chronic HIV. His management has presented numerous challenges. While his viral load is well controlled to undetectable levels, and his CD4$^+$ count is greater than 500 cells/mm$^3$, he continues to engage in unsafe sexual practices. Today he comes to clinic with a new skin condition. He reports the acute onset of a rash on both arms. It appeared rather suddenly and does not hurt or itch or present any symptoms. Physical examination reveals a bilateral macular eruption to both arms extending almost to the elbow. The ACNP suspects:

    a.  Gonorrhea
    b.  Disseminated herpes zoster
    c.  Kaposi's sarcoma
    d.  Syphilis

10. A 54-year-old male presents to an urgent care center where he is seen by an ACNP. He has no significant past medical history. He has been experiencing severe flank pain for two days, is currently afebrile, and denies urgency or hesitancy. A urinalysis reveals less than 10 WBC/HPF. The most appropriate diagnostic evaluation to assess the cause of his symptoms would be a:
    a.  Stone collection and analysis
    b.  CBC and metabolic panel
    c.  Thorough history and physical examination
    d.  CT scan

11. You are the ACNP in the emergency department. A middle-aged male presents with excruciating flank pain and nausea with vomiting. The KUB reveals a 4 mm diameter ureteral stone. Based on this finding the appropriate action would be:

    a.  Referral for lithotripsy
    b.  Intravenous pyelography (IVP) to assess for obstruction
    c.  Analgesia and hydration
    d.  Serum and urine blood tests to assess stone mineral type

12. A 38-year-old male presents with a sudden onset of renal insufficiency. His history and physical examination are benign, with the exception of a new diagnosis within the last year of hypertension. Renal artery stenosis is suspected. Which of the following statements is not true regarding renal artery stenosis?

    a.  Renal artery stenosis is progressive and can lead to loss of renal function.
    b.  Compensatory, contralateral hypertrophy may temporarily maintain renal function.
    c.  Renal artery stenosis should be suspected when hypertension develops in a previously normotensive client.
    d.  A negative captopril test is diagnostic of renal artery stenosis.

13. The ACNP is evaluating a 61-year-old male patient who presented to the emergency department for an evaluation of chest pain that ultimately was diagnosed as gastroesophageal reflux disease (GERD). However, during a thorough review of systems, the patient revealed that for approximately 1 year he has had a persistent, progressive difficulty voiding. He often gets up during the night to void, and sometimes has to wait a long time for the stream to begin. He sometimes feels as though he cannot empty his bladder. Which of the following will provide the most useful diagnostic information?

    a.  A prostate specific antigen (PSA)
    b.  A postvoid residual catheterization
    c.  A digital rectal examination
    d.  A urinalysis

14. Mr. P. is a 73-year-old male who presents to the outpatient clinic with frequency, urgency, and leakage of urine for the past month. Which of the following should not be included in the differential diagnosis?

a. Prostate cancer
b. Benign prostatic hypertrophy
c. Acute bacterial prostatitis
d. Epididymitis

15. A 32-year-old female presents with fever, nausea and vomiting, and back pain. Upon examination, the ACNP appreciates costovertebral angle (CVA) tenderness, and the urinalysis reveals leukocytes and bacteria. Which of the following features is anticipated in the patient's history?

a. New onset of vigorous sexual activity
b. A urinary tract infection 10 days ago for which she took TMP/SMX
c. Just completed a course of antibiotics for sinus infection
d. A history of nephrolithiasis last summer

## ◘ ANSWERS AND RATIONALE

1. **(c)** Pyelonephritis is an upper urinary tract infection of the renal parenchyma. Characteristic findings include flank, low back, or abdominal pain, fever, chills, and white blood casts seen on urinalysis. Cystitis, or lower urinary tract infection, does not typically cause back pain or fever in otherwise healthy young adults; urinary symptoms are the presenting feature. Gonorrhea is usually asymptomatic in women, and discovered during cervical screening. While bacterial vaginosis may produce white blood cells that are seen in urine, the other urinary symptoms are not present as it is not an infection of the urinary tract (McPhee & Papadakis, 2009).

2. **(d)** This patient does not have syphilis, and does not require repeat testing unless he engages in high-risk behavior. The VDLR is a highly sensitive screening test, which means that there are no false negatives; a negative result means the patient does not have syphilis.

However, it is not highly specific, which means false positive is possible. Positive screening tests need to be confirmed with a highly specific confirmatory test. The FTA-Abs is a highly specific confirmation test that does not produce false positives; if the FTA-Abs is negative, the patient does not have syphilis, and if it is positive, the patient does have syphilis. The combination of the two test results reported here is interpreted as negative. The patient clearly is subject to some other circumstance that produced a false positive screening VDRL (CDC, 2007; Wallach, 2006).

3. **(d)** Urine sodium and fractional excretion of sodium ($FE_{Na+}$) determination can differentiate a prerenal from an intrarenal cause of oliguria. Prerenal failure is due to diminished glomerular perfusion pressure; there is no nephron damage present. The conservation of sodium is maintained and urine sodium levels are low (< 20 mmol/dL) and the $FE_{Na+}$ is low (< 1%). In intrarenal failure, nephron damage has occurred, thus impairing the normal absorption and secretion ability of the tubules. Urine sodium levels are elevated (> 40 mmol/dL) and the $FE_{Na+}$ is elevated (> 3%), indicating impairment in sodium reabsorption due to tubular damage (Marino, 2007; Wallach, 2006).

4. **(b)** Patients are often asymptomatic until the late stages of CKD (stages 4 and 5) due to the compensatory ability of functioning nephrons. Stage 2 CKD can represent a wide range of nephron loss in either direction of 50%. Nephron loss is irreversible. While stage 1 CKD does produce a compensatory increase in GFR, by the time the patient progresses to stage 2, GFR is always below baseline (Fauci, 2007).

5. **(d)** Postrenal failure occurs due to mechanical or functional urine flow obstruction. If untreated, postrenal failure

can progress to intrarenal failure with the time frame being dependent on the degree, mechanism, and duration of obstruction. Reversing hypo-perfusion is characteristic of prerenal failure, and intrarenal failure damages basement membrane (Cooper, 2007).

6. **(c)** HPV is the most common STI in the US and is viral. There are numerous subtypes, some of which are causative of genital warts and others of cervical malignancy. Chlamydia is the most common *bacterial* sexually transmitted infection in the United States (CDC, 2007).

7. **(d)** Gonorrhea is a sexually transmitted bacterial infection that is a leading cause of infertility in US females, but not the leading cause. Gonorrhea is often asymptomatic in women but can produce dysuria and vaginal discharge: however, many women do not know they are infected unless screened. All contacts should be treated and cases reported to the health department. Uncomplicated gonorrhea is treated with any one of several single-dose antibiotic regimens and does not typically require 14–28 days of treatment (CDC, 2007).

8. **(a)** Herpes is a viral, sexually transmitted disease with no cure. It is associated with painful genital lesions that are spread through direct contact with virus-containing fluid or active lesions. Primary infection virtually always results in an outbreak within 6–8 weeks of infection; subsequent outbreaks tend to be less severe and preceded by a prodrome. While the male outbreak is typically visible and external, female outbreaks may be intravaginal and not apparent to the patient. In this case, IgM indicates recent primary infection (within 6–8 weeks) for the male, and IgG indicates remote infection (may be years) for the female. Because of the wide variability in terms of outbreak, it is very possible that the female was infected prior to this relationship and was unaware. This presentation unfortunately does happen and does not imply infidelity. While the couple may have issues to resolve, "a" is the best choice of those provided. Antiviral therapy has no impact on transmission if both partners are infected, and antiviral treatment does not cure (CDC, 2007; McPhee & Papadakis, 2009).

9. **(d)** This rash represents the classic presentation of secondary syphilis, which occurs approximately 6 weeks after infection. The patient should immediately be screened for syphilis. Gonorrhea produces genitourinary symptoms, with uncommon dissemination to joints to produce a gout-like manifestation. Herpes zoster is characterized by a vesicular eruption, and Kaposi's sarcoma may have a similar morphology, but does not typically present as sudden and bilateral nor does it typically occur in the well-controlled, immunocompetent patient (Burns & Breathnach, 2010; CDC, 2007).

10. **(d)** The most likely diagnosis is renal calculi. More common in men with an average age of onset greater than 30 years, renal calculi often present with flank pain that is usually seen with increasing intensity, radiating downward to the groin or over the abdomen. Consequently, the most appropriate diagnostic study would be a CT scan. Stone analysis may aid with the determination of interventions, but it will not diagnose the problem. A CBC and metabolic panel will not offer diagnostic information for this symptom complex. While a thorough history and physical examination is always the starting point for any differential, renal calculi is not a clinical diagnosis and should have imaging confirmation (Cooper, 2007).

11. **(c)** Analgesia and hydration are important initial treatment measures for renal calculi. If the stone is less than 6 mm in diameter, observation for passage for a 4-week period is advised. Referral to a urologist is indicated if the stone does not pass within a 4-week period. If the stone is obstructing urine outflow or is accompanied by infection, removal is indicated. Lithotripsy is a more aggressive intervention indicated for stones greater than 6 mm. IVP is not indicated at this point as the diagnosis is made. Serum and urine assessment will not provide stone type; in any event, assessment of stone type is not an intervention (McPhee & Papadakis, 2009).

12. **(d)** Renal artery stenosis can be diagnosed with a positive captopril test. A captopril test is positive when an exaggerated increase in plasma renin activity results from the administration of captopril. Uncorrected, RAS may lead to loss of renal function and should always be considered as an underlying cause of secondary hypertension in a previously normotensive patient. As with most organ systems, compensatory changes by the other kidney may delay symptom onset, delaying diagnosis until the disease is quite advanced (Fauci, 2007).

13. **(c)** This symptom complex is highly suspicious for benign prostate hypertrophy (BPH). The patient needs a thorough digital rectal examination to assess the gland. PSA is not specific, and a normal PSA does not preclude diagnosis. A postvoid residual volume may or may not be elevated at any given time; a normal result does not preclude diagnosis. Urinalysis is not an indicator of prostate function (McPhee & Papadakis, 2009).

14. **(d)** Prostate cancer, benign prostatic hypertrophy, and acute bacterial prostatitis all would be considered in the differential diagnosis of an elderly male with frequency, urgency, and leakage of urine. Severe scrotal pain, relieved by elevation, and fever would be characteristic of epididymitis and is much less common in this age group (McPhee & Papadakis, 2009).

15. **(b)** This presentation is suggestive of acute pyelonephritis, a common cause of which is the ascension of an inadequately treated lower urinary tract infection. Vigorous sexual activity would more likely precipitate a lower urinary tract infection such as cystitis, and recent antibiotic therapy would likely precipitate a yeast infection. While a history of nephrolithiasis would increase risk for recurrent nephrolithiasis, this patient is febrile with leukocytes in urine, which suggests an infectious process (CDC, 2007; McPhee & Papadakis, 2009).

## ◘ REFERENCES

Burns, T., Breathnach, S., Cox, N., & Griffiths, C. (2010). *Rook's textbook of dermatology* (8th ed.). Malden, MA: Wiley-Blackwell.

Centers for Disease Control and Prevention (CDC) (2006). Sexually transmitted diseases treatment guidelines. *Morbidity and Mortality Weekly Report, 55* (No. RR-11), 1–94.

Cooper, D. H., Krainik, A. J., Lubner, S. J., & Reno, H. E. L. (2007). *The Washington manual of medical therapeutics* (32nd ed.). Philadelphia, PA: Lippincott, Williams, & Wilkins.

Fauci, A. S., Braunwald, E., Kasper, D. L., Hauser, S. L., Longo, D. L., Jameson, J. L., & Loscalzo, J. (Eds.). (2008). *Harrison's principles of internal medicine* (17th ed.). New York: McGraw-Hill.

Marino, P. L. (2007). *The ICU book* (3rd ed.). Philadelphia, PA: Lippincott, Williams, & Wilkins.

McPhee, S. J., & Papadakis, M. A. (Eds.). (2009). *Current medical diagnosis and treatment* (48th ed.). New York: McGraw-Hill.

Seidel, H. M., Ball, J. W., Dains, J. E., & Benedict, G. W. (2006). *Mosby's guide to physical examination* (6th ed.). St. Louis: Mosby, Inc.

US Preventive Services Task Force (USPSTF). (2007). *The guide to clinical preventive services: Recommendations of the United States Preventive Services Task Force.* Retrieved on March 28, 2010 from http://www.ahrq.gov. clinic/pocketgd.pdf.

Wallach, J. (2007). *Interpretation of diagnostic tests* (8th ed.). Philadelphia, PA: Lippincott, Williams, & Wilkins.

# 12

# Musculoskeletal Disorders

*Lynn A. Kelso*

## Select one best answer to the following questions.

1. A 37-year-old male is complaining of severe right ankle pain and swelling that began suddenly 2 hours ago. Vital signs are BP 108/76 mm Hg, heart rate 114 bpm, respiration 18 bpm, and temperature 97.6°F. Past medical history is significant for multiple ankle sprains. He has no known drug allergies (NKDA) and his only medication is atorvastatin. Definitive diagnosis will be made with:

   a. Urine cultures
   b. Bilateral ankle radiographs
   c. Joint fluid aspirate
   d. Serum uric acid level

2. Typical early radiographic features of degenerative joint disease (DJD) include:

   a. Joint space narrowing
   b. Soft tissue swelling
   c. Thick, dense subchondral bone
   d. Punched-out bony erosions

3. A 36-year-old female is complaining of burning pain and tingling that radiates up her forearm. She first experienced symptoms a few months ago and noticed them when she woke up in the morning. Now symptoms occur more frequently throughout the day. The ACNP knows that the best test for confirming the clinical diagnosis will be:

   a. Tinel's test
   b. Carpal compression test
   c. Upper extremity radiographs
   d. Left upper extremity (LUE) electromyography

4. The ACNP is called to the emergency department to assess a patient who is being evaluated by the trauma service. The patient was found unresponsive at the site of a single-car motor vehicle accident on a remote road; no one knows precisely how long he was unconscious. He appears to be drug intoxicated; drug screen is pending. Among other injuries, he is found to have bilateral tibial fractures, and the paramedics report that both legs were bent in an

unusual position under his body when they found him. The ACNP will be alert for:

a. Hypoxia and tachypnea
b. Shiny, tense, nonpitting edema
c. Blackish discoloration of the tips of the toes
d. Acute lymphedema in the popliteal region

5. A 52-year-old male is complaining of severe lower back pain. The most important diagnostic tool for evaluating his complaint is a:

a. Thorough history and physical
b. Complete set of spinal radiographs
c. CT of the abdomen
d. MRI of the spine

6. A 73-year-old female with a history of osteoarthritis is complaining of fatigue, lightheadedness, and dyspnea on exertion. Her history is significant only for the osteoarthritis that has been successfully managed with ibuprofen 800 mg tid. Along with serum electrolytes and an ECG, the evaluation should include a(n):

a. Echocardiogram
b. Sputum C&S
c. Guaiac stool
d. Chest radiograph

7. The ACNP is managing a patient with severe bilateral knee pain due to osteoarthritis. He has not been responsive to either high-dose acetaminophen or high-dose ibuprofen. The nurse practitioner knows that curative treatment will probably include:

a. Opioid management
b. Surgical intervention
c. TNF inhibitors
d. Intra-articular steroid injections

8. A 54-year-old male being treated for renal insufficiency is on furosemide 80 mg IV bid. He was awakened during the night with severe pain in his right foot localized to the first and second metatarsophalangeal joints. The therapy of choice would be:

a. Indomethacin and $MSO_4$
b. Indomethacin and colchicine
c. Colchicine and allopurinol
d. Methylprednisolone and $MSO_4$

9. A 63-year-old female was admitted to the hospital with severe back pain. Her past medical history is significant for chronic atrial fibrillation, hypertension, and a hysterectomy for cervical cancer at age 51. An abdominal source of back pain has been ruled out. You then order a:

a. Myelogram
b. Lumbar puncture
c. Spinal radiograph
d. MRI of the spine

10. A 49-year-old male is complaining of severe neck pain with frequent muscle spasms, which increase in intensity any time that he coughs. Physical examination reveals upper extremity DTR of +1 and decreased bilateral forearm sensation. The ACNP should order:

a. Ice compresses bid
b. Physical therapy
c. Ibuprofen 800 mg q12h
d. Cervical traction and bedrest

## ◻ ANSWERS AND RATIONALE

1. **(c)** This patient presents with acute, monoarticular joint inflammation, the most common cause of which is gout. Initial evaluation typically includes a serum uric acid level, but definitive diagnosis is made with joint fluid analysis and visualization of crystals. While radiographic changes are typical with chronic gout, it is not a sensitive diagnostic marker in first presentation (McPhee & Papadakis, 2009).

2. **(a)** Joint space narrowing is the earliest radiographic feature of DJD, and in later disease there is virtually no space left between two bones. Later disease

is also characterized by thickened bone and sometimes the development of bony nodules. Soft tissue swelling is characteristic of rheumatoid arthritis, and punched-out erosion is suggestive of late stage gout (Fauci, 2007).

3. **(d)** These symptoms are consistent with carpal tunnel syndrome, a median neuropathy at the wrist. Tinel's test is a classic, but not very sensitive clinical assessment in which tapping the skin over the flexor retinaculum produces symptoms over the nerve distribution. A negative result does not rule out carpal tunnel. The carpal compression test (Durkin's test) has also been proposed as a clinical assessment in which pressure is placed over the palm for 30 seconds to produce symptoms. Radiography does not provide an assessment of nerve function and does not contribute to diagnosis. Electromyography provides an assessment of nerve conduction (Fauci, 2007; Seidel *et al.*, 2006).

4. **(b)** This patient is at high risk for compartment syndrome, including trauma and prolonged pressure on the lower extremities. Upon awakening he would complain of severe pain, particularly when the extremity is stretched; however, before he awakes, tense edema may develop as tissues swell. Black toes represent a much later manifestation of loss of blood flow. Hypoxemia and tachypnea may represent any variety of problems, but compartment syndrome is more compelling given the limited history. Lymph node enlargement is not an acute, trauma-related event (Marino, 2007).

5. **(a)** The most common mistake made when evaluating patients with lower back pain is not obtaining an adequate history and physical examination. Lower back pain is a manifestation of many processes, and a thorough history and physical examination can lead the

evaluation in specific directions. Most commonly, low back pain is due to either musculoskeletal strain or radiculopathy, and imaging is not indicated (Tollison, 2002).

6. **(c)** Osteoarthritis is frequently treated with nonsteroidal anti-inflammatory drugs (NSAIDs). These need to be used with caution in the elderly because gastrointestinal bleeding associated with the use of NSAIDs is increased in this population. The patient's symptoms may represent anemia, and GI bleeding should be ruled out. An echocardiogram is not indicated in the absence of other cardiac risk factors. Sputum for C&S is almost never contributory unless obtained during a bronchoscopy, and the chest radiograph is not indicated with this history (Cooper, 2007).

7. **(b)** Osteoarthritis that does not respond to NSAIDs will likely require surgical replacement for optimal management. Chronic opiod use is not desirable due to risk of dependency, and is only used in nonsurgical candidates. TNF inhibitors are not useful for OA; they are used in RA. Intra-articular steroids are used for symptom management, but do not constitute curative therapy (McPhee & Papadakis, 2009).

8. **(d)** The patient is exhibiting symptoms of acute gout, which can be exacerbated with hyperuricemia precipitated by diuretics. Although NSAIDs are frequently used to treat acute gout, they should be avoided or used with extreme caution in patients with renal insufficiency. The best treatment option would be steroids, which often provide dramatic symptomatic relief. Opioids may also be required to relieve pain (McPhee & Papadakis, 2009).

9. **(c)** Postmenopausal osteoporosis frequently becomes clinically evident about 10 years after menopause. The greatest loss is with trabecular bone,

which frequently leads to vertebral crush fractures. This would be evident with spinal radiographs (Cooper, 2007).

10. **(d)** A herniation of the cervical disks into the spinal canal causes pain that radiates to the arms. There are frequently muscle spasms associated with the pain, and it is aggravated by maneuvers that increase intra-abdominal pressure, such as coughing or sneezing. Decreased deep tendon reflexes may be seen as well as weakness in the forearms. Conservative therapy, including cervical traction and bedrest, is usually successful. Although ibuprofen may help to alleviate pain, the dose given is not appropriate and should be 200 to 400 mg every 4 to 6 hours (Tollison, 2002).

## ◻ REFERENCES

Cooper, D. H., Krainik, A. J., Lubner, S. J., & Reno, H. E. L. (2007). *The Washington manual of medical therapeutics* (32nd ed.). Philadelphia, PA: Lippincott, Williams, & Wilkins.

Fauci, A. S., Braunwald, E., Kasper, D. L., Hauser, S. L., Longo, D. L., Jameson, J. L., & Loscalzo, J. (Eds.). (2008). *Harrison's principles of internal medicine* (17th ed.). New York: McGraw-Hill.

Marino, P. L. (2007). *The ICU book* (3rd ed.). Philadelphia, PA: Lippincott, Williams, & Wilkins.

McPhee, S. J., & Papadakis, M. A. (Eds.). (2009). *Current medical diagnosis and treatment* (48th ed.). New York: McGraw-Hill.

Seidel, H. M., Ball, J. W., Dains, J. E., & Benedict, G. W. (2006). *Mosby's guide to physical examination* (6th ed.). St. Louis: Mosby, Inc.

Tollison, C. D., Satterthwaite, J. R., & Tollison, J. W. (2002). *Practical pain management.* (3rd ed.). Philadelphia, PA: Lippincott, Williams, & Wilkins.

Wallach, J. (2007). *Interpretation of diagnostic tests* (8th ed.). Philadelphia, PA: Lippincott, Williams, & Wilkins.

# 13

# Common Problems in Acute Care

*Candis Morrison*

## Select one best answer to the following questions.

1. G. Y. is a 52-year-old male who is 6 hours postemergency appendectomy. His temperature has risen from 97.5°F preoperatively to 100.5°F postoperatively. The most likely cause of his fever is:

   a. Atelectasis
   b. Pneumonia
   c. IV site infection
   d. Wound infection

2. The ACNP is evaluating a 77-year-old female who is in the emergency room with a chief complaint of fever of 102.4°F. The physical exam is significant only for some mild confusion. Urinalysis and chest radiograph are negative, and cultures are pending. A CBC reveals a mild normocytic anemia, but the WBC differential is within normal limits. The next step in the assessment should include:

   a. A thorough review of medications
   b. An MRI of the head
   c. A CT of the abdomen
   d. An erythrocyte sedimentation rate (ESR)

3. Fever is a common indicator of infection in the acute care setting, and when other indices of infection are present, it is very appropriate to begin broad spectrum antibiotics empirically while cultures are pending. All of the following conditions are indications for empiric antibiotic therapy in febrile patients except:

   a. Temperature > 100.5°F
   b. Hemodynamic instability
   c. Neutropenia
   d. Concomitant use of systemic corticosteroids

4. Which of the following represents the most accurate statement with respect to around-the-clock antipyretic use in the management of fever?

   a. Routine use of antipyretics is never indicated as fever has important diagnostic and prognostic value in all patients.
   b. Routine use of antipyretics is indicated in the management of fever of unknown origin when no cause is found after a full, inpatient diagnostic evaluation.

c. Routine use of antipyretics is indicated when the patient does not have sufficient reserves to withstand the metabolic costs of fever.

d. Routine use of antipyretics should not extend beyond 96 hours in any patient due to the risk of hepatorenal toxicity with high serum levels of acetaminophen, ibuprofen, or ASA.

5. R. L. is a 34-year-old male patient just returned from the operating room (OR) for repair of a hiatal hernia. The patient is morbidly obese, and the surgery was complicated by an iatrogenic pneumothorax and a nicked spleen. Consequently, there was a significant amount of fluid loss and the patient requires a closely supervised recovery. The ACNP anticipates which type of acid-base imbalance?

    a. Respiratory acidosis
    b. Respiratory alkalosis
    c. Metabolic acidosis
    d. Metabolic alkalosis

6. An 82-year-old female is transferred from the long-term care facility for a transfusion of packed red blood cells (PRBC) for a hemoglobin of 9.2 g/dL attributed to anemia of chronic disease. A basic metabolic panel reveals a serum Na$^+$ of 131 mEq/L. Unfamiliar with the patient, the ACNP orders a serum osmolality, which is 280 mOsm/L. Which of the following is the most appropriate action?

    a. A urine Na$^+$ should be assessed to evaluate renal losses.
    b. No further action is indicated as this is pseudohyponatremia.
    c. A TSH should be drawn as hypothyroidism is a common cause of mild hyponatremia.
    d. A chest radiograph should be performed to evaluate for congestive heart failure.

7. A 24-year-old male presents to the emergency department complaining

that his hands and feet are tingling and numb. He is clearly agitated, and history reveals that he takes escitalopram 20 mg daily. Aside from some mild tachycardia and tachypnea the physical exam is within normal limits. The next appropriate action by the ACNP would be to:

    a. Consider a CT of the head
    b. Order alprazolam 1 mg p.o.
    c. Explain that his current symptoms are a function of his anxiety
    d. Obtain a 12-lead ECG

8. The ACNP recognizes that who among the following patients would most likely exhibit a normal gap acidosis?

    a. A patient with type 1 diabetes mellitus (DM) who is currently in ketoacidosis
    b. A patient who presents with an acute mental status change who is diagnosed with ethylene glycol intoxication
    c. A patient with chronic obstructive pulmonary disease who developed an acute exacerbation
    d. A patient with dialysis-dependent renal failure

9. Which of the following conditions is associated with neutropenia?

    a. Temporal arteritis
    b. Cushing's disease
    c. Felty's syndrome
    d. Systemic lupus erythematosus

10. A 49-year-old patient with human immune deficiency virus (HIV) has a CD4$^+$ count of 300 cells/mm$^3$. He presents with fatigue, tachypnea, and a low-grade temperature. The ACNP anticipates which presentation on the chest radiograph?

    a. Diffuse bilateral infiltrates
    b. Lobar consolidation
    c. Increased retrosternal airspace
    d. Flattened diaphragm

11. A patient with chronic respiratory acidosis secondary to COPD is admitted

with acute respiratory failure. The ACNP knows that the ventilator settings should maintain some element of hypercapnia because:

a. Dropping the $CO_2$ too quickly will arrest his respiratory drive
b. It will protect him from oxygen toxicity that can occur with $FIO_2 > 60\%$
c. His baseline $HCO_3-$ will be elevated due to COPD
d. Hypercapnia is the primary respiratory driver in COPD patients

12. A 19-year-old college student presents to the emergency department complaining of lightheadedness, anxiety, numbness in her hands and feet, and numbness around her mouth. She has a history of panic disorder and takes escitalopram daily for anxiety. Chest radiograph is normal and her arterial blood gases reveal a low $PaCO_2$. The first intervention indicated to correct her acid base disorder is to:

a. Administer $O_2$ at 6 L/min via nasal cannula
b. Administer sodium bicarbonate IV
c. Have her rebreathe into a paper bag
d. Have her take rapid shallow breaths

13. A patient with a long history of congestive heart failure has been on loop diuretics for 6 years. He recently experienced 6 days of nausea and vomiting that he attributed to food poisoning. Today he presents with weakness, lethargy, hypotension, and decreased skin turgor. ABG reveals a pH of 7.47 and an elevated serum bicarbonate. Therapy should include infusion of:

a. $HCO_3-$
b. $D_5W$
c. Colloids
d. Normal saline

14. In an apparent suicide attempt, a 22-year-old female ingested 16 acetaminophen tablets 4 hours ago. Her serum acetaminophen level is 250 µg/mL. The appropriate antidote for this overdose is:

a. Naloxone
b. Flumazenil
c. Activated charcoal
d. N-acetylcysteine

15. A 29-year-old paraplegic has been admitted urgently for management of autonomic dysreflexia. A central line has been placed. Four days later the patient develops a temperature of 102.7°F and the central line insertion site appears erythematous and tender to touch. This patient most likely has line sepsis due to:

a. *Pseudomonas aeruginosa*
b. *Staphylococcus epidermidis*
c. *Proteus mirabilis*
d. *Streptococcus pneumoniae*

16. An unidentified male is brought to the emergency department by friends. He is stuporous and confused. On examination he has pinpoint pupils and is hypotensive. He has track marks on both arms. Shortly after admission, he loses consciousness and experiences respiratory arrest. The ACNP would order:

a. Diazepam
b. Haloperidol
c. Flumazenil
d. Naloxone

17. A patient is brought to the emergency department status postoverdose of an unknown substance. On initial examination her pupils are pinpoint. Her heart rate is 46 bpm and her BP is 90/40 mm Hg. She is drooling copiously and has been incontinent of urine and stool. The ACNP recognizes all of these findings as a classic _____ overdose.

a. Opioid
b. Amphetamine
c. Benzodiazepine
d. Cholinergic

18. While reviewing morning labs on an 82-year-old male patient being treated for urinary tract infection, the ACNP appreciates an abnormal serum Ca++ of 13.7 mEq/L. When evaluating the patient, the ACNP may expect to find that the patient:

a. Is having involuntary twitches of skeletal muscle
b. Is lethargic as compared to his baseline
c. Has developed a prolonged p-r interval on ECG assessment
d. Has a coincident rise in serum Cl⁻

19. A 19-year-old college sophomore is admitted to the emergency department. History reveals that he consumed 15 12-oz beers over the course of 2 hours while participating in a party drinking game. Vital signs on admission include a temperature of 37.2°C, heart rate of 112 bpm, respiration of 10 bpm, and BP of 90 mm Hg palpable. He is difficult to arouse. He weighs approximately 70 kg. Which of the following treatment plans is most appropriate?

a. Administer disulfiram intravenously
b. Allow the patient to "sleep it off" in a holding room
c. Insert a nasogastric (NG) tube and evacuate gastric contents
d. Admit for CNS and respiratory monitoring

20. T. J. is a 23-year-old male who presents with a 4-day-old abscess in his left forearm. The arm is tender, warm, indurated, and erythematous. He complains of fatigue, but otherwise is without systemic symptoms. The mass is fluctuant and well encapsulated, with no tracking. There is no inflammation of proximal lymph nodes, and the patient is afebrile. Treatment must include:

a. Incision and drainage
b. Elevation and compression
c. Systemic antibiotics
d. Topical antibiotics

21. A 34-year-old male is brought to the emergency department with a 4 cm clean, deep laceration on the dorsum of his foot, sustained by a lawn mower blade. His past health history is negative for chronic illness. In preparation for suturing, it would be appropriate to:

a. Soak the foot in 100% betadine solution and debride wound edges
b. Shave the area around the laceration and soak in 10% betadine solution
c. Assess motor and sensation of the toes
d. Clean the periphery with 1% betadine solution and then irrigate

22. J. S. is a 59-year-old female patient with a history of cirrhosis. She is hospitalized for surgical debridement of an infected wound, and has developed hyponatremia. The serum osmolality is 261 mOsm/L, and the patient has clinical signs and symptoms of volume contraction. The ACNP suspects that the underlying cause of hyponatremia is:

a. Rising ammonia levels
b. Overuse of loop diuretics
c. Sepsis
d. Retention of free water

23. J. S. is a 50-year-old male brought to the emergency department after sustaining burns to his entire right arm, right leg, and the right side of the thorax and abdomen. These are all second- or third-degree burns. What is the best estimate of percentage of his body that is burned?

a. 27%
b. 36%
c. 45%
d. 54%

24. A 35-year-old male patient presents to the urgent care clinic. He is in significant pain and admits that he was working in the crawl space under his home when he felt a deep pain in his right upper arm. Upon examination the area is mildly edematous and painful to

touch. There does not appear to be a foreign body, but there is clearly a small hole that appears to be a penetrating injury. The patient has no idea when he last had a tetanus shot. The ACNP would order:

a. Tetanus toxoid 0.5 cc
b. Tdap 0.5 cc and TIG (tetanus immune globulin) 250 U
c. Td 0.5 cc and TIG (tetanus immune globulin) 250 U
d. TIG (tetanus immune globulin) 250 U

25. A 43-year-old male is admitted to the medical intensive care unit (MICU). Vital signs are as follows: temperature 97.1°F, heart rate 80 bpm, respiration 20 bpm, and BP 150/104 mm Hg. He is lethargic and confused. Chest examination reveals bilateral crackles and an $S_3$ heart sound. He has 4 cm of jugular venous distention (JVD) bilaterally. His deep tendon reflexes (DTRs) are decreased throughout and he has a urine output of less than 15 mL per hour. Laboratory evaluation demonstrates a serum Na$^+$ of 132 mEq/L, a serum K$^+$ of 3.2 mEq/L, a serum osmolality of 245 mosm/L, and a urine Na$^+$ of greater than 20 mEq/L. This clinical picture is most consistent with hyponatremia due to:

a. Failure of a primary organ
b. Hypothyroidism
c. Iatrogenic fluid overload
d. Excess sodium and fluid losses

26. Enteral feedings are begun on a patient s/p CVA with swallowing abnormalities. Within 24 hours the patient develops diarrhea characterized by several brown liquid stools. The ACNP knows that the most appropriate intervention would be to:

a. Slow down the feeding and titrate up very gradually
b. Begin concomitant use of loperamide (Imodium)
c. Change the solution used for feeding
d. Observe for 72 hours before making any adjustments

27. Your head-injured patient has had 400 mL per hour urine output over the last 4 hours. The specific gravity is 1.002. A recent chemistry panel revealed a serum glucose of 96 mg/dL. Which diagnosis is most consistent with this clinical scenario?

a. Prolactinoma
b. Diabetes insipidus
c. Syndrome of inappropriate antidiuretic hormone
d. Addison's disease

28. An 85-year-old patient is admitted for acute mental status change. According to the caretaker she is normally alert and oriented, and her only real problem is limited mobility due to severe osteoarthritis. The caretaker reports that yesterday she became acutely confused, did not know what day it was, and did not want to get dressed before sitting in her outdoor lawn chair. The ACNP knows that the most likely cause of her symptoms is:

a. Dementia
b. Dehydration
c. Delirium
d. Drug effects

29. A 43-year-old patient was admitted to the medical intensive care unit (MICU) with symptoms of intense thirst and polyuria (reportedly ingesting > 10 L per day). He also complains of dizziness, muscle cramps, headaches, weight loss, and fatigue. On examination he has dry mucous membranes, poor skin turgor, and postural hypotension. Pre-admission laboratory evaluation demonstrated a serum sodium of 152 mEq/L, with a serum osmolality of 300 mOsm/L. Urine osmolality was less than 10 mOsm/L and urine specific gravity was also low. Urine glucose was negative. The ACNP suspects which of the following etiologic features:

a. A cardiac dysrhythmia
b. A pituitary abnormality
c. An adrenal tumor
d. Recent immobility

30. You are admitting a patient with refractory hypotension and a decreasing level of consciousness. The basic metabolic panel reveals a $Na^+$ of 129 mEq/L, $K^+$ of 6.1 mEq/L, $Cl^-$ of 103 mEq/L, $CO_2$ of 24 mEq/L, BUN of 22 mg/dL and creatinine of 1.2 mg/dL. The glucose is 61 g/dL. This constellation of electrolyte abnormalities is consistent with:

    a. Pseudohyponatremia
    b. Diuretic excess
    c. Growth hormone excess
    d. Adrenocortical insufficiency

31. The ACNP is evaluating a patient who is scheduled for surgical repair of a hernia. During the examination a mass is identified in the left hypochondrum. The mass pulsates with heart rate. The patient is otherwise stable. The next appropriate step would be to:

    a. Cancel the surgery
    b. Consult vascular surgery
    c. Obtain bilateral upper extremity blood pressure assessments
    d. Obtain a CT scan of the abdomen

32. An important complication of inadequately treated acute hyponatremia would be:

    a. Central diabetes insipidus
    b. Cerebral dehydration
    c. Cerebral embolus
    d. Cerebral edema

33. A 79-year-old male is brought to the ED complaining of shortness of breath of 1 day's duration and a 2-day history of nausea, vomiting, and weakness. He has been unable to pass urine for the past 18 hours. Past medical history is positive for atrial fibrillation, COPD, and benign prostatic hypertrophy (BPH). Medications include digoxin and coumadin. Vital signs include a temperature of 100.7°F, heart rate of 126 bpm, respiration of 28 bpm, BP of 118/60 mm Hg, and an $O_2$ saturation of 92%. 2L of $O_2$ are administered per nasal cannula. He is attached to the cardiac monitor, which demonstrates sinus tachycardia with prolonged p-r intervals and wide QRS complexes that are irregularly placed. As suspected, his $K^+$ is elevated at 7.5 mEq/L. Which underlying condition is the most likely cause of the hyperkalemia?

    a. Metabolic acidosis secondary to chronic hypoperfusion
    b. Respiratory acidosis secondary to COPD
    c. Reduced potassium excretion secondary to BPH
    d. Metabolic alkalosis secondary to vomiting

34. A positive nitrogen balance is a good indication that which of the following therapeutic interventions is working?

    a. Total parenteral nutrition (TPN)
    b. Lactulose enemas
    c. Fluid restriction
    d. Bedrest

35. A 65-year-old alcoholic male is found to have a serum $Ca^{++}$ of 6.5 mEq/dL. He is carefully questioned regarding symptoms of the disorder and reports generalized muscle cramps and paresthesias around his lips. Which additional laboratory value would you need to rule out a calcium abnormality?

    a. Albumin
    b. Globulin
    c. Glucose
    d. Potassium

36. A 72-year-old woman presents complaining of nausea, polyuria, and constipation. Her muscles are weak upon examination and she exhibits depressed deep tendon reflexes. She has been supplementing her diet with calcium antacids in an effort to prevent osteoporosis. Her serum $Ca^{++}$ is 11 mEq/dL. Serum albumin is normal. In an effort to correct the calcium you would begin treatment with:

    a. Stopping the calcium supplements
    b. Normal saline with loop diuretics
    c. Colloids and magnesium
    d. Normal saline and insulin

37. Patients on ACE inhibitors should be monitored for which two adverse effects of these drugs?

    a. Hyperkalemia and proteinuria
    b. Hypokalemia and thrombocytopenia
    c. Nephrotoxicity and congestive heart failure
    d. Atrial fibrillation and hyponatremia

38. A 63-year-old is brought to the urgent care center by her daughter. It is reported that over the course of the past 2 days she has become increasingly anxious. She is awake all night and seems drowsy during the day. On examination she is irritable, anxious, and pacing around the room. She denies a problem with her memory, though her daughter states that she is extremely forgetful. Her past medical history is negative, with the exception of a CVA 3 years ago. Physical examination is unremarkable. She scores 20 on a Folstein mini-mental status examination and is having extreme difficulty attending. The most common cause of delirium in an elderly patient is:

    a. Hypoxia
    b. Drug ingestion
    c. Electrolyte imbalance
    d. Infection

39. The ACNP is counseling an 18-year-old patient recovering from a humoral fracture. Due to the nature of her injury, he suspects domestic violence, which the patient has denied. The patient has a one-year-old child with cerebral palsy, and her husband is unemployed. The ACNP should ask specifically about:

    a. Family support
    b. Accessibility of counseling services
    c. Previous injuries
    d. Access to firearms

40. An 84-year-old woman is hospitalized for a hip fracture. Throughout the hospitalization it becomes clear that she has some deficits in short-term memory and executive function. The ACNP suspects:

    a. Delirium
    b. Vascular dementia
    c. Alzheimer's dementia
    d. Lewy body dementia

41. A 32-year-old male is admitted with the diagnosis of acute confusional state. Symptom onset was sudden and associated with visual hallucinations and psychomotor restlessness. Physical examination reveals tachycardia, dilated pupils, and diaphoresis. An important component of his initial evaluation is a:

    a. Dexamethasone suppression test
    b. Toxicology screen
    c. 12-lead ECG
    d. Pulse oximetry

## ◘ ANSWERS AND RATIONALE

1. **(a)** Differential diagnosis of postoperative fever can be narrowed down by considering the time relationship of the onset of the fever to the surgery. Atelectasis and volume contraction are the two most common causes of fever during the first 24 hours postoperatively secondary to decreased inflation of alveoli and blood loss during surgery. When infection occurs as a consequence of operation, it is typically at least 72 hours after the procedure (Doherty, 2009).

2. **(a)** Fever is a common presenting complaint in the elderly and is most commonly attributed to infection. However, this patient does not have any indicators of infection, and noninfectious causes must be considered. Drug fever is among the leading causes of noninfectious fever in this age group, as the average elderly adult takes six prescription and two over-the-counter medications. More invasive imaging and laboratory studies may be ordered later in the evaluation, but a review of the drug list is quick, noninvasive,

and should be performed immediately (McPhee & Papadakis, 2009).

3. **(a)** Most fever is well tolerated. Mild elevations only require fluid replacement, and a temperature of 100.5°F does not warrant empiric antibiotics. Empiric antibiotic therapy is indicated in cases with high concurrent risk factors, such as comorbid immunosuppression (e.g., neutrenia or concomitant high-dose steroid use) and in situations in which the patient is at risk for poor outcomes, such as hemodynamic instability (McPhee & Papadakis, 2009).

4. **(c)** Routine use of antipyretics is generally more a case of provider convenience than evidence-based care. Fever does have diagnostic and prognostic value with respect to its timing, duration, and 24-hour fluctuation. When possible, fever should progress unmedicated so that the body can maximize the therapeutic effects of fever, and the provider can evaluate fever features to aid in diagnosis and management. However, fever does have extensive metabolic costs in terms of caloric burn and myocardial oxygen demand. When the patient has significant cardiopulmonary disease or lacks fat stores, the risks of fever outweigh the benefits and around-the-clock use is indicated. While frequent, long-term use of common antipyretics can be hepatorenal toxic, if the patient requires them for more than 96 hours, they should be continued (Fauci, 2008).

5. **(d)** Metabolic alkalosis is the most common acid-base abnormality in the postoperative patient, and occurs as a consequence of fluid loss. In the absence of chloride, the most abundant extracellular anion, the kidney will compensate by reabsorbing another negatively charged ion, $HCO_3^-$. This produces a metabolic alkalosis alkalsis that will resolve with the infusion of normal saline solution (NSS). As the kidneys resume reabsorption of chloride,

$HCO_3^-$ will be excreted and normal balance restored (Doherty, 2009).

6. **(b)** The patient has normotonic hyponatremia (pseudohyponatremia) as evidenced by the normal osmolality. This is not unusual in older patients as a consequence of mild hyperlipidemia. If the serum osmolality were low, then further assessment would be indicated to rule out CHF, liver, or renal failure. Urine $Na^+$ is evaluated in patients with hypotonic hyponatremia and a low volume status (McPhee & Papadakis, 2009).

7. **(c)** This young man is experiencing "stocking glove paresthesia," which is a common consequence of respiratory alkalosis. Hyperventilation produces respiratory alkalosis, which leads to these transient distal symptoms. The first action is to reassure the patient that his symptoms do not indicate a dangerous condition, and that if he can slow his breathing, they will resolve. Many times the symptoms are improved by having the patient breathe into a paper bag. While benzodiazepines may be required, the first action is reassurance. Aggressive diagnostics are not indicated in this scenario (Ferri, 2006).

8. **(d)** The evaluation of anion gap compares the difference between the number of positively and negatively charged ions in serum. As a function of the laws of electroneutrality, the body maintains a limited gap, usually less than 20. However, in the setting of acute acidotic states, this balance is temporarily lost, and the patient is said to have a high gap acidosis. Normal gap acidoses are characteristic of chronic acidotic states; patients with acute acidoses will typically have high gaps. Gap is calculated as $(Na^+ + K^+) - (Cl^- + HCO_3^-)$. Some references only use $Na^+$ and $Cl^-$ as the parameters, but the principle is unchanged; under normal circumstances, there should not be a significant gap between positive and

negative charges in serum. When that gap occurs, the acidosis is acute (Cooper, 2007).

9. **(c)** Felty's syndrome is a rare consequence of immune neutropenia, seen in some patients with seropositive rheumatoid arthritis. Temporal arteritis and systemic lupus erythematosus are autoimmune conditions characterized by a normal white blood cell differential. Cushing's syndrome is an adrenocortical excess that increases neutrophils (McPhee & Papadakis, 2009).

10. **(a)** Pneumocystis pneumonia is the most common opportunistic infection in patients with HIV, and this clinical scenario is consistent with it. Typical radiographic presentation of pneumocystic pneumonia includes bilateral diffuse infiltrates, much like other atypical pathogens. Lobar consolidation would be expected in a more typical pneumonia such as streptococcus. Increased retrosternal airspace and flattened diaphragm are more consistent with COPD (Mandell, 2005).

11. **(c)** Patients with COPD have chronic $CO_2$ retention and compensatory metabolic $HCO_3^-$ retention. If the $CO_2$ is normalized, the excess $HCO_3^-$ will produce a state of uncompensated metabolic alkalosis. For this reason, COPD patients who are ventilated should not be ventilated to a normal $CO_2$, but to their baseline. Hypercapnia does not protect from oxygen toxicity. Hypercapnia is the respiratory driver in all humans, but it is not a reason to maintain hypercapnia (Marino, 2007).

12. **(c)** Hyperventilation is the likely etiology for these symptoms, particularly in an individual with an anxiety/panic disorder. The rapid respirations produce respiratory alkalosis, which results in palpitations and "stocking glove paresthesia." Treatment is directed toward the underlying cause. In acute hyperventilation syndrome from anxiety,

rebreathing into a paper bag will increase $PaCO_2$. If unsuccessful, sedation may be required (Cooper, 2007).

13. **(d)** This clinical picture is consistent with metabolic alkalosis from volume contraction. Patients maintained on diuretics therapy may become unstable when other circumstances alter their normal fluid balance, such as nausea and vomiting or decreased fluid intake. This disorder should respond to saline as the therapy includes correction of the extracellular volume deficit. Adequate amounts of 0.9% NaCl and KC1 should be administered as the patient is likely to be hypochloremic, hyponatremic, and hypokalemic. Diuretics should also be discontinued pending normalization (Cooper, 2007).

14. **(d)** The specific antidote for acetaminophen is N-acetylcysteine. It is dosed at 140 mg/kg and is most effective when administered in the first 16 hours after ingestion; however, it should be given up to 24 hours after ingestion. The antidote is recommended if the serum level exceeds the toxic line on the nomogram for prediction of hepatotoxicity following acute overdose. Naloxone is the antidote for an opiate overdose, and flumazenil the antidote for benzodiazepine overdose. Activated charcoal is used to bind ingested toxins, but has not demonstrated utility in acetaminophen overdose (McPhee & Papadakis, 2009).

15. **(b)** The two most common causes of line sepsis in the immunocompetent patient are *staphylococcus aureus* and *staphylococcus epidermidis*, the gram positive organisms that colonize the skin. Pseudomonas should be considered in those with immunocompromise or other risk factors for pseudomonal infection. Streptococcus is possible but less common on skin, and proteus is unlikely unless there is a known exposure (Doherty, 2009).

16. **(d)** This case is suggestive of narcotic overdose, probably heroin. Treatment is naloxone 2 mg IV. Results are evident within 2 minutes and are quite dramatic. Diazepam and haloperidol have sedative properties and should not be given to this patient under any circumstances. Flumenazil will not reverse opiate overdose as it is indicated for benzodiazepine overdose (Ma *et al.*, 2004; Katzung, 2009).

17. **(d)** This patient is exhibiting cholinergic—i.e, parasympathetic—signs such as those seen secondary to organophosphate poisoning, with insecticides. These act as anticholinesterase agents and produce classic exaggeration of cholinergic symptoms, e.g., bradycardia, hypotension, pupil constriction, salivation, and bowel and bladder activation. The antidote for this poisoning is atropine 0.5 to 2 mg IV. Atropine physiologically blocks acetylcholine. Opiate poisoning presents with dilated pupils and urinary retention. Amphetamine overdose produces cardiovascular escalation, such as hypertension and tachycardia, with dilated pupils. Benzodiazepine overdose presents as altered mental status and hypotension, but no lacrimation or salivation. (Ma, 2004; McPhee & Papadakis, 2009; Katzung, 2009).

18. **(b)** Normal serum $Ca^{++}$ is between 8.5 and 10 mEq/L. The patient is hypercalcemic, which presents as decreasing level of consciousness and may lead to death if not corrected. Twitching would be seen in hypocalcemic states. A prolonged p-r interval is more likely due to drug toxicities, but may be seen in hyperkalemia. There is not a coincident rise in $Cl^-$ (McPhee & Papadakis, 2009).

19. **(d)** This patient reveals signs of acute intoxication. A 12-oz bottle of beer raises the blood alcohol level by 25 mg/dL in a 70 kg person. Lethal blood levels are in the range from 350 to 900 mg/dL. This patient requires close monitoring for acute alcohol overdosage leading to respiratory depression, seizures, and/or shock. Disulfiram is contraindicated in acute intoxication, but is used to deter drinking in cases of alcohol abuse. Evacuating gastric contents would not be helpful at this point (Ma, 2004).

20. **(a)** The lesion described in the scenario is one that requires incision and drainage. Absent systemic symptoms or risk factors for complicated resolution, an isolated lesion does not require administration of antibiotics, either topically or systemically (Doherty, 2009).

21. **(c)** First and foremost before taking any action with wound, including anesthetizing the area, a neurovascular check should be performed. If there is any sensory or motor deficit, it is likely that a nerve has been damaged and this should be addressed before suturing the wound. Following neurovascular assessment, preparing the wound for repair should include anesthesia with 1% lidocaine and irrigation. There is no evidence that needles can spread bacteria beyond wound margins, so most wounds should be anesthetized before cleaning. A 1% betadine solution can be safely applied to wounds and retains its bactericidal activity at this concentration. Dirty wounds should be irrigated. Research has demonstrated that soaking cannot penetrate beyond 1.5 mm of tissue and significant contamination may result. Shaving can increase the wound infection rate. (Doherty, 2009; Ma *et al.*, 2004).

22. **(b)** Because the patient has clinical findings of volume contraction, she is losing salt as well as water, with a disproportionately high loss of salt. This suggests a history of diuretic overuse, as diuretics promote renal excretion of ions, and will do so even as volume falls. If she were retaining free water she would have symptoms of volume overload. Ammonia levels are not

directly related to hyponatremia. Sepsis may produce electrolyte and other metabolic abnormalities, but not the specific hypotonic, hypovolemic, hyponatremia described here (Doherty, 2009; McPhee & Papadakis, 2009).

23. **(c)** The "rule of nines" is commonly used for estimating burn size in adults. Each arm is 9%, each leg 18%. The entire thorax and abdomen (anterior and posterior) is 36%. Since one half was affected, you add 18% + 9% + 18% = 45%. First degree burns are not included in these calculations (Ma *et al.*, 2004).

24. **(b)** Because the patient does not know his tetanus immunization status, he must be protected from immediate infection with TIG. However, TIG will not confer long-term immunity, so he also needs the vaccine that will promote immune development for the next several years. Current recommendations are for one dose of Tdap in place of Td for adults up to age 64. Then a Td booster should be given every 10 years (Cooper, 2007; USPSTF, 2007).

25. **(a)** This patient has hypotonic hyponatremia and clear evidence of fluid overload. His sodium is diluted as a function of free water retention. This is most often due to failure of either the heart, liver, or kidney; his examination suggests acute congestive heart failure. Treatment will include free water restriction and diuresis with replacement of salt-rich fluid. Hypothyroidism causes a mild hyponatremia but not the hypertension and decreased urine output (McPhee & Papadakis, 2009).

26. **(a)** Most tube feeding solution is very hyperosmolar and initially draws water into the gut, producing diarrhea. The appropriate management is to decrease the amount of feed and reintroduce gradually so that the gut can adjust to the osmolarity of the feeding. Daily antidiarrheals are a last resort, and changing the solution is only necessary if the patient cannot tolerate the contents of the solution. Allowing the diarrhea to progress for several days may dehydrate an already compromised patient, and is not necessary since there are alternatives (Doherty, 2009).

27. **(b)** Classic signs and symptoms of DI include diuresis of very dilute urine with normal serum glucose. The history of head injury is a clue to the diagnosis (Marino, 2007).

28. **(c)** This is a classic presentation of delirium. The most common cause of delirium in an elderly patient is infection, and this patient should have urinalysis, urine cultures, and a chest radiograph as part of the initial assessment. Dementia does not have such an acute global onset. There is no indication that she has taken any new medications or increased doses, and there are no indicators of dehydration (Ferri, 2006).

29. **(b)** This clinical picture is consistent with diabetes insipidus, a condition in which the patient is either not producing ADH or the kidney is not responding to it. Most common causes include damage to the posterior hypothalamus caused by head injury, tumor, surgery, etc. A progressive headache is consistent with an evolving tumor. Cardiac dysrhythmia would not increase urine output, and while an adrenal tumor may cause changes in fluid retention depending upon tumor type, it would not produce this volume of urine output. Immobility ultimately decreases urinary output (Doherty, 2009; Marino, 2007).

30. **(d)** Acute adrenal insufficiency is an emergent condition caused by insufficient adrenal hormones. Lack of cortisol would cause low to low-normal blood sugar. The lack of aldosterone results in the inability of the renal tubule to reabsorb sodium and excrete potassium, thereby resulting in hyponatremia and

hyperkalemia (Parrillo & Dellinger, 2008).

31. **(d)** The mass as described is suspicious for an abdominal aortic aneurysm, and the diagnosis needs to be confirmed with a CT scan. Comparison of upper extremity blood pressures will not contribute to the assessment at this point. While hernia surgery will be cancelled and vascular surgery will be consulted if the patient has a confirmed aneurysm, the next step at this point is to confirm the diagnosis (McPhee & Papadakis, 2009).

32. **(d)** Patients with symptomatic, severe, acutely developed hyponatremia require emergency treatment. $Na^+$ is the primary extracellular ion, and when $Na^+$ levels are low, there is a significant risk that hypoosmolar serum will result in an intracellular shift of water, causing cerebral edema and subsequent neurologic toxicity. This may progress to seizures, obtundation, coma, and cerebral herniation (Ferri, 2006).

33. **(c)** Renal potassium excretion will increase in response to serum hyperkalemia, therefore transcellular shifts are generally mild. Serum potassium concentration rarely exceeds 6.0 mEq/L unless there is a simultaneous reduction in renal potassium excretion. This patient's history of BPH and his inability to void have produced a postobstructive renal failure with subsequent potassium retention. Mild respiratory acidosis would cause no significant rise in serum potassium concentration, nor would acute lactic acidosis (Fauci, 2007).

34. **(a)** A positive nitrogen balance is an indicator that the patient is taking in more protein than is nutritionally required, and it is a marker of TPN efficacy. TPN is usually begun when patients need nutritional support, characterized by a breakdown of protein stores and negative nitrogen balance. When the balance becomes positive, this suggests adequate nutrition. Otherwise healthy patients typically have a neutral balance, but in those on TPN, a positive balance is desirable (Doherty, 2009).

35. **(a)** The depressed level of serum calcium must be correlated with the simultaneous concentration of serum albumin. Albumin is the principle calcium-binding protein. Approximately 60% of circulating calcium is bound to albumin, so if albumin is low, the binding ratio is skewed. Low albumin is correlated with depressed calcium in a ratio of 0.8 to 1 mg of calcium to one gram of albumin. The history of alcoholism could predispose to a hypoalbuminemic state (McPhee & Papadakis, 2009).

36. **(a)** This clinical picture is consistent with the milk-alkali syndrome associated with ingestion of calcium supplements used for osteoporosis. In this syndrome, massive calcium and Vitamin D ingestion can cause hypercalcemic nephropathy. Excretion of sodium is accompanied by excretion of calcium. The first intervention is to stop the ingestion of supplements. If hypercalcemia persists, inducing calcium excretion by giving saline with furosemide is the treatment of choice for hypercalcemia. Calcium-rich fluid is diuresed and replaced with calcium-poor fluid, thus diluting serum calcium. If the patient is unresponsive to this therapy, dialysis may be indicated (Ferri, 2006).

37. **(a)** ACE inhibitors may cause hyperkalemia through inhibiting the secretion of aldosterone triggered by angiotensin II. Proteinuria may occur and even lead to nephrotic syndrome and renal failure. The practitioner needs to monitor serum $K^+$ and urine protein for these potential effects (Katzung et al., 2009).

38. **(d)** Delirium is an acute symptom that typically represents a reversible abnormality external to the CNS. In the elderly, infection is the most common cause. All elderly patients with delirium should be assessed for infection. Other causes include hypoxia, drug toxicity, depression, and electrolyte abnormality (McPhee & Papadakis, 2009).

39. **(d)** The leading cause of morbidity and mortality in this age group is accidental. The patient's home environment is characterized by multiple stressors, and violence is suspected. With primary attention to safety, the ACNP should assess for access to firearms (McPhee & Papadakis, 2009).

40. **(c)** The subtle presentation of symptoms suggests dementia rather than delirium. Alzheimer's dementia is the most common type, and the age of the patient presents a risk factor. Vascular dementia is more common in those with other vascular disease and risk factors, and Lewy body dementia has a more rapid, deterioriation course (Fauci, 2007).

41. **(b)** Substance or alcohol withdrawal is the most common cause of delirium in young adults in the general hospital setting and is a treatable cause of delirium. A toxicology screen is required to confirm the diagnosis and specifically identify the substance (McPhee & Papadakis, 2009).

## ◘ REFERENCES

Cooper, D. H., Krainik, A. J., Lubner, S. J., & Reno, H. E. L. (2007). *The Washington manual of medical therapeutics* (32nd ed.). Philadelphia, PA: Lippincott, Williams, & Wilkins.

Doherty, G. (2009). *Current surgical diagnosis and treatment* (13th ed.). New York: McGraw-Hill.

Fauci, A. S., Braunwald, E., Kasper, D. L., Hauser, S. L., Longo, D. L., Jameson, J. L., & Loscalzo, J. (Eds.). (2008). *Harrison's principles of internal medicine* (17th ed.). New York: McGraw-Hill.

Ferri, F. F. (2006). *Practical guide to the care of the medical patient* (7th ed.). Philadelphia, PA: Mosby.

Katzung, B. G., Masters, S. B., & Trevor, A. J., (Eds.). (2004). *Basic and clinical pharmacology* (11th ed.). New York: McGraw-Hill.

Ma, O. J., Cline, D. M., Tintinalli, J. E., Kelen, G. D., & Stapczynski, J. S. (2004). *Emergency medicine manual* (6th ed.). Philadelphia, PA: McGraw-Hill Professional.

Mandell, G. L., Bennett, J. E., & Dolin, R. (2005). *Principles and practice of infectious diseases* (6th ed.). London: Churchill Livingstone.

Marino, P. L. (2007). *The ICU book* (3rd ed.). Philadelphia, PA: Lippincott, Williams, & Wilkins.

McPhee, S. J., & Papadakis, M. A. (Eds.). (2009). *Current medical diagnosis and treatment* (48th ed.). New York: McGraw-Hill.

Parrillo, J., & Dellinger, R. (Eds.). (2008). *Critical care medicine: Principles of diagnosis and management in the adult* (3rd ed.). St. Louis: Mosby, Inc.

US Preventive Services Task Force (USPSTF). (2007). *The guide to clinical preventive services: Recommendations of the United States Preventive Services Task Force.* Retrieved on March 28, 2010 from http://www.ahrq.gov. clinic/pocketgd.pdf.

# 14

# Shock States/ Trauma

*Candis Morrison*

## Select one best answer to the following questions.

1. A 29-year-old female is brought to the emergency department by paramedics, status postgunshot wound to the abdomen following a domestic dispute. Paramedics estimate that she has lost two liters of blood. Her pulse is weak at 140 bpm and her blood pressure is palpable at 50 mm Hg. Skin is cool and extremities are cyanotic. Neck veins are completely flat. The chest is clear, and heart sounds are weak. To prevent irreversible shock-related complications while preparing her for the operating room, it is important to immediately infuse:

   a. Isotonic crystalloids through a short, large-bore IV
   b. Colloids at a rate of 3 to 4 times the volume deficit
   c. Sodium bicarbonate to prevent metabolic acidosis
   d. Broad spectrum antibiotics to prevent sepsis

2. A 32-year-old woman is 1-day postoperative cardiac transplant for cardiomyopathy. Her mediastinal tube has been draining normally. Vital signs at 8 a.m. reveal a temperature of 98.6°F, heart rate of 124 bpm, respiration of 28 bpm, and BP of 86/50 mm Hg. Her skin is cold and clammy. There is 9 cm of JVD at 45 degrees and crackles in both bases. The ACNP knows that appropriate interventions for this patient will not include:

   a. Aggressive isotonic fluid infusion
   b. Decreasing preload with nitroglycerin
   c. Increasing contractility with inotropic agents
   d. Supporting oxygenation

3. The condition of a patient in the ICU has just deteriorated. He was being treated for pulmonary embolus, but despite aggressive supportive therapy, his blood pressure has dropped to 60/30 mm Hg and his heart rate has increased to 145 bpm. You observe that his jugular veins are visibly distended. Which type of shock is most consistent with this history and these findings?

a. Hypovolemic
b. Obstructive
c. Distributive
d. Cardiogenic

4. You are called to the emergency department to admit a patient who is reportedly in shock. His blood pressure is palpable at 70 mm Hg, and his heart rate is 160 bpm. On examination his extremities are pink and warm. The ACNP knows that effective management must include:

a. Vasopressors
b. Inotropes
c. Colloids
d. Antibiotics

5. A. P. is a 52-year-old patient with a history of HIV and Hodgkin's disease. She has completed her first cycle of chemotherapy and presents for admission for her second cycle. She is complaining of lethargy, weakness, anorexia, and fever. Her total white blood cell count is 500/μL with an absolute neutrophil count of 230/μL, and hemoglobin is 8 g/dL. Her temperature is 103.6°F, heart rate 136 bpm, respiration 32 bpm, and BP is palpable at 60 mm Hg. She is admitted, and a pulmonary artery catheter is placed. Her cardiac output is 11 mL/min and the pulmonary artery wedge pressure is 5 mm Hg. Arterial blood gases reveal the following: pH 7.26, $PaCO_2$ 25 mm Hg, $HCO_3^-$ 16 mEq/L, and $PaO_2$ 64 mm Hg. This clinical picture is most consistent with which form of shock?

a. Hypovolemic
b. Anaphylactic
c. Septic
d. Neurogenic

6. A 47-year-old construction worker is transported to the emergency department by his co-workers. They say that they do not know what happened, but that he appeared to be gasping and then became unconscious. His blood pressure is 90/54 mm Hg but falling. His pulse is 125 bpm. Physical examination reveals a large stinger protruding from his neck. The ACNP knows that his falling blood pressure is related to:

a. Hypoxia secondary to bronchoconstriction
b. Compensatory catecholamine release
c. Reflex release of adrenocortical hormone
d. IgE mediated vasodilation

7. Aggressive fluid resuscitation is indicated in all of the following shock states except:

a. Hypovolemic
b. Obstructive
c. Cardiogenic
d. Distributive

8. M. M. is a 59-year-old male patient in the ICU being managed for an acute shock state. His cardiac pressures reveal a CVP of 14 mm Hg, PAOP 5 mm Hg, SVR of 1620 dynes $\times$ sec/cm$^5$ and a cardiac index of 1.2 L/min. The ACNP suspects which of the following underlying causes?

a. Pulmonary embolus
b. Congestive heart failure
c. Trauma
d. Anaphylaxis

9. A patient is brought to the emergency department after a motor vehicle accident. He is diagnosed with respiratory distress. On examination his breath sounds are decreased on the right, and there is hyperresonance to percussion over the left lower lobe. Shortly after arrival his left breath sounds disappear, and he begins to evidence signs of shock—tachycardia, hypotension, and confusion. As the ACNP you immediately:

a. Order a chest radiograph to determine need for a chest tube
b. Order a chest CT to assess for pneumothorax

Shock States/Trauma **93**

c. Insert a needle in the second right intercostal space anteriorly

d. Intubate immediately to prevent hypoxia

10. Neurogenic shock is a type of distributive shock that occurs in response to spinal cord injury above the level of $T_6$. As a result of the underlying neurogenic dysfunction, expected assessment findings would include:

a. Hypotension and bradycardia

b. Peripheral vasoconstriction and hyperthermia

c. Hypotension refractory to fluid infusion

d. Hypotension refractory to vasopressors

11. A 27-year-old female is transported to the trauma emergency department after being evacuated from an industrial accident in which she was trapped in an imploded building. She is alert and responsive upon arrival; however, she was unconscious when paramedics reached the accident scene. She is wearing a cervical collar and requests that it be removed. The ACNP knows that the collar may be safely removed after:

a. A complete neurologic examination of the extremities

b. C-1 to C-7 are radiographically visualized and declared normal

c. Glasgow coma score is $\geq 11$

d. Head CT reveals no evidence of cranial bleed

12. A 40-year-old female is transported to the emergency department following rescue from a multiple-car accident. She had to be extracted from her seat belt and was trapped tightly between the seat and the steering wheel. The patient is not alert enough to give any history, but an eyewitness account is that she drove directly into the car in front of her without slowing down. While considering diagnostic peritoneal lavage, the ACNP knows that which of

the following is a contraindication to this diagnostic procedure?

a. Pelvic fracture

b. Previous abdominal surgery

c. Falling hematocrit

d. Lower chest injury

## ◻ ANSWERS AND RATIONALE

1. **(a)** This patient is in hypovolemic shock due to rapid loss of blood. Shock in the setting of trauma is always presumed to be hypovolemic, and his clinical findings support that impression. The mainstay of management of hypovolemic shock is rapid restoration of vascular volume. Animal models have demonstrated that, during the early phase of hypovolemic shock, cardiac output and arterial pressure can be returned to normal by administration of fluids in the first 90 minutes even when more than 40% of blood volume was rapidly lost. When isotonic fluids are used, it is necessary to infuse three to four times the estimated lost volume. Smaller quantities of colloids are required to restore circulating blood volume. Bicarbonate is not indicated unless the pH is less than 7.1. Antibiotics will be infused prophylactically, but in the immediate phase isotonic fluids are most critical to preserve life (ACS, 2008; Doherty, 2009).

2. **(a)** This patient exhibits clinical indications of pump failure and cardiogenic shock secondary to decreased contractility. The primary treatment will include inotropic agents, and additional therapies may include preload reduction and controlled fluid support, but aggressive fluid resuscitation is not indicated. Oxygen support is always indicated for treatment of shock (Bongard et al., 2008; Cooper, 2007).

3. **(b)** The history of pulmonary embolus is consistent with obstructive shock, in which an external pressure on the

ventricle precludes filling. Volume is trapped in the atria leading to jugular venous distention. Cardiogenic shock also produces venous distention as a consequence of high atrial pressures, but the history would be significant for risk factors for pump failure. Distributive shock is characterized by widespread vasodilator and maldistribution of vascular contents; JVD does not occur. Similarly, hypovolemic shock, as the name implies, is characterized by a significant decrease in intravascular volume (Bongard *et al.*, 2008; McPhee & Papadakis, 2009).

4. **(d)** In hypovolemic and cardiogenic shock, the circulating concentrations of catecholamines and angiotensins rise, producing vasoconstriction or cold shock. Distributive shock is manifested in an opposite manner as a consequence of the release of endotoxin and endogenous vasodilators. These produce peripheral vasodilation, or warm shock, in which the patient has warm extremities despite hypotension. Distributive shock is also known as high output shock. The most common cause of distributive shock is sepsis, which requires antibiotic therapy for successful management. Vasopressors may be indicated, but it is appropriate to first restore blood pressure with volume. Colloids are indicated in some circumstances, but crystalloids would be the first fluid attempt (Bongard, 2008; Parrillo & Dellinger, 2008).

5. **(c)** This patient's history and hemogram demonstrate risk for septic shock. Microbial pathogens trigger events involving exogenous and endogenous mediators that cause diffuse vascular inflammation, intravascular coagulation, and decreased vascular smooth muscle tone leading to loss of regulation of cardiac output and its distribution (Parrillo & Dellinger, 2008; Mandell, 2005).

6. **(d)** Anaphylaxis produces a widespread release of IgE that produces simultaneous bronchoconstriction and vasodilation. The patient wheezes and is unable to respire; at the same time diffuse vasodilation occurs resulting in a distributive shock state as the entire vascular bed dilates. Catecholamine release does occur, but it does not cause hypotension. Hypoxia may occur, but it does not produce vasodilation—in fact, it would promote vasoconstriction absent the maladaptive vasodilation. Adrenocorticotropic hormone release will occur later to promote return to hemostasis (Cooper, 2007; Ferri, 2006).

7. **(c)** A primary concern in managing the shock patient is maintaining a blood pressure adequate to perfuse the vital organs until the cause of the shock can be identified and treated. Fluid resuscitation is indicated in every form of shock, because the more fluid that goes into the left ventricle, the more that will be delivered into arterial circulation. However, in cardiogenic shock, fluid volume status is not the problem. Paradoxically, patients may appear to be in fluid overload, and additional large volumes of fluid may actually decrease effectiveness of contraction and output. Therefore, modest fluid infusion is indicated, and aggressive fluid resuscitation is not indicated in cardiogenic shock (ACS, 2008).

8. **(a)** These cardiac pressures suggest obstructive shock, in which some external pressure on the ventricle (e.g., pneumothorax, pulmonary embolus, or cardiac tamponade) restricts ventricular filling. CVP pressures are elevated due to fluid back-up, but PAOP (PCWP) is low due to low volume in the ventricle. The peripheral arterial bed constricts to try and increase pressure, so SVR increases. Cardiac index is low as there is decreased volume for ejection. Cardiogenic shock would produce a high PAOP, and hypovolemic and distributive

shocks would result in a low CVP. Additionally, distributive shock would produce a low SVR (Bongard, 2008; Parrillo & Dellinger, 2008).

9. **(c)** This patient evidences signs of obstructive shock due to tension pneumothorax. This develops when a puncture in the visceral pleura functions as a valve, allowing air to be drawn into the pleural space during inspiration and preventing it from escaping during expiration. The resulting rise in pleural pressure compresses the heart and great veins, thus obstructing cardiac output. Management must be directed at restoration of the pressure gradient for venous return. Air in the chest should be evacuated quickly either through a chest tube or by inserting a large bore needle between two ribs. Imaging is not indicated as the patient is acutely unstable and the cause is readily apparent from clinical assessment (Marino, 2007).

10. **(a)** Neurogenic shock is characterized by severe autonomic dysfunction. This will produce hypotension and relative bradycardia, making it different from other shock states, which usually produce tachycardia until just before death. Peripheral vasodilation and hypothermia are also a consequence of autonomic dysfunction (Schreiber, 2009).

11. **(b)** Injury to the cervical spine must be assumed to be present whenever consciousness is disturbed secondary to trauma. Five to ten percent of such patients will have a major cervical injury. Absolute immobilization of the C-spine is critical in patients presenting after trauma with even minor abnormalities of mental status, significant head or facial injuries, or other symptoms suggestive of cervical injury. Immobilization should be maintained until three-view radiologic visualization of C-1 to C-7 is complete and determined to be normal (Ma *et al.*, 2004; Wilkinson, 2001).

12. **(b)** Nonpenetrating trauma to the abdomen should be considered when the patient is subjected to a crush injury or acceleration/deceleration injury. Seat belts may exacerbate the risk. This patient cannot provide any information, and recognizing that the physical examination is negative in up to 20% of patients with nonpenetrating injury, a DPL should be considered. Indications include unexplained abdominal pain, injury to lower chest, pelvic fracture, abdominal trauma with altered mental status, and hypotension with falling hematocrit. Contraindications include previous abdominal surgery, pregnancy, and operator inexperience (Doherty, 2009; Wilkinson, 2001).

## ◼ REFERENCES

American College of Surgeons (ACS). (2008). *Advanced trauma life support course for doctors.* Chicago: Author.

Bongard, F., Sue, D. Y., & Vintch, J. R. E. (2008). *Current diagnosis and treatment: Critical care* (3rd ed.). New York: Lange Medical Books/McGraw-Hill.

Cooper, D. H., Krainik, A. J., Lubner, S. J., & Reno, H. E. L. (2007). *The Washington manual of medical therapeutic*s (32nd ed.). Philadelphia, PA: Lippincott, Williams, & Wilkins.

Darovic, G. O. (2002). *Hemodynamic monitoring: Invasive and noninvasive clinical application* (3rd ed.). Philadelphia, PA: Saunders.

Doherty, G. (2009). *Current surgical diagnosis and treatment* (13th ed.). New York: McGraw-Hill.

Fauci, A. S., Braunwald, E., Kasper, D. L., Hauser, S. L., Longo, D. L., Jameson, J. L., & Loscalzo, J. (Eds.). (2008). *Harrison's principles of internal medicine* (17th ed.). New York: McGraw-Hill.

Ma, O. J., Cline, D. M., Tintinalli, J. E., Kelen, G. D., & Stapczynski, J. S. (2004). *Emergency medicine manual* (6th ed.). Philadelphia, PA: McGraw-Hill Professional.

Marino, P. L. (2007). *The ICU book* (3rd ed.). Philadelphia, PA: Lippincott, Williams, & Wilkins.

McPhee, S. J., & Papadakis, M. A. (Eds.). (2009). *Current medical diagnosis and treatment* (48th ed.). New York: McGraw-Hill.

Parrillo, J., & Dellinger, R. (Eds.). (2008). *Critical care medicine: Principles of diagnosis and management in the adult* (3rd ed.). St. Louis: Mosby, Inc.

Schreiber, D. M. (2009). Spinal cord injuries. *Emedicine.* Retrieved on October 20, 2009 from http://emedicine.medscape.com/article/793582-overview.

Wilkinson, D. A., & Skinner, M. W. (2001). *Primary trauma care manual.* World Health Organization. Retrieved on November 1, 2009 from http://www.steinergraphics.com/surgical/manual.html.

# 15

# Pain and Immobility

*Lynn A. Kelso*

## Select one best answer to the following questions.

1. A 62-year-old male is recovering from surgical repair of a large abdominal aortic aneurysm (AAA). His recovery has been prolonged by numerous complications including sepsis and respiratory failure. He is much better now, and his pain management is being changed from continuous maintenance to prn administration. While educating for optimal pain management, the ACNP advises him that:

   a. It is best that he try to tolerate increasing time intervals without medication.
   b. As he increases ambulation pain medication will be less necessary.
   c. Taking medication before pain reaches maximum intensity will provide the greatest control.
   d. Narcotic dose can be decreased by adding a benzodiazepine.

2. After weaning a patient from vecuronium, an $MSO_4$ drip, and lorazepam, the ACNP attempts to assess his neurologic function. He remains sedated and is only responsive to noxious stimuli. The appropriate action would be to:

   a. Order a head CT scan
   b. Give 0.2 mg flumazenil IV
   c. Order an EEG
   d. Wait and reassess in 24 hours

3. A 21-year-old male, status postcholecystectomy, is complaining of incisional pain. He has an order for intermittent IM $MSO_4$. The ACNP knows that according to step_____ of the World Health Organization (WHO) pain management guideline, nonsteroidal anti-inflammatories should be added to the narcotic regimen to maximize pain control.

   a. 1
   b. 2
   c. 3
   d. 4

4. It is important that patients begin ambulating as soon as possible following a period of bedrest for either medical or surgical management. This is because immobility can increase the risk of all of the following except:

a. Deep vein thrombosis
b. Pneumonia
c. Paralytic ileus
d. Congestive heart failure

5. J. T. is a 37-year-old healthy male who sustained bilateral femur fractures during a recreational vehicle accident. He is confined to bed pending stabilization and surgical repair. He has a foley catheter in place and comments on the amount of urine that it is draining. The ACNP tells him that when a healthy patient becomes suddenly immobile, urine output:

   a. Decreases as glomerular blood flow declines with immobility
   b. Increases due to increased venous return of blood and subsequent increased flow to renal afferent
   c. Decreases markedly with the abrupt decline in activity but then resumes as the body adjusts to the change in level of activity
   d. Increases significantly for 4–5 days but then decreases if bedrest is prolonged.

6. You are evaluating a 39-year-old patient with diabetes who is complaining of bilateral foot pain. There are no lesions or wounds on either foot, and pulses are present with doppler. He is experiencing minimal relief from oxycodone HCl. The most appropriate action would be to:

   a. Discontinue the oxycodone and begin pregabalin
   b. Add ibuprofen to the oxycodone
   c. Increase the dose of oxycodone and prescribe Vicodin for breakthrough pain
   d. Begin prednisone, then taper off the oxycodone

7. A 54-year-old patient with colon cancer is recovering from insertion of a diverting PEG tube. Her disease is terminal, and her baseline pain level is increasing almost daily. She is currently taking 80 mg of long-acting morphine bid and is still having breakthrough pain. The ACNP knows that the next appropriate step in pain management for this patient is:

   a. To discontinue the morphine and begin a Fentanyl patch
   b. Begin a continuous morphine infusion
   c. Add regularly scheduled NSAIDs to the regimen
   d. Begin a morphine infusion and add a benzodiazepine

8. A 78-year-old male being treated for prostate cancer is on the following medications: Digoxin 0.25 mg p.o. q.d.; nifedipine SR 90 mg q.d.; oxycodone HCl 2 p.o. q4h. Although he states he has no other pain, he is complaining of abdominal cramping and has not had a bowel movement in 3 days. The ACNP recognizes that:

   a. The nifedipine is likely slowing down the smooth muscle of the gut and should be discontinued.
   b. Constipation is a frequent visceral response to pain and would likely improve if pain control were optimized.
   c. The constipation is probably due primarily to the immobility, and the patient should be encouraged to ambulate.
   d. A common consequence of long-term narcotic management is constipation.

9. A 73-year-old female has been on bedrest for 3 weeks at home. When attempting to get out of bed, she became lightheaded and had to be helped back to bed by her caregiver. To prevent this the caregiver should:

   a. Increase the patient's fluid intake
   b. Position the patient as close to upright as possible tid
   c. Do passive range-of-motion exercises tid
   d. Sit the patient for 5 minutes prior to standing.

10. You are the new ACNP who has joined an internal medicine practice. You are assigned as primary provider for a panel of patients previously covered by one of the partner physicians. One of the more challenging cases is a 47-year-old obese male who has been maintained on Lortab for chronic back pain for the last 3 years. He currently takes Lortab 10-mg tablets 3 to 4 times daily and presents for a refill. The ACNP tells him that chronic multiple daily Lortabs is not good practice for a variety of reasons, and surprisingly, the patient agrees to try an alternate regimen. An appropriate first change in medication management would be to:

    a. Introduce a daily AED
    b. Reduce the Lortab to 2 times daily
    c. Convert to a once daily long acting opiate
    d. Add an NSAID

11. In a patient on bedrest, which of the following will increase the risk for developing a deep vein thrombosis (DVT)?

    a. Increased body mass index (BMI)
    b. Hypertension
    c. Thrombophilia
    d. Liver disease

12. An 82-year-old male has been on self-prescribed bedrest since the death of his wife. His son is concerned and has brought him into the hospital. The patient's past medical history is unremarkable, and he is currently on no medications. He denies any pain. The next step in his care should include:

    a. A mental status examination
    b. A Geriatric Depression Scale
    c. Zoloft 50 mg q.d.
    d. Cranial imaging

## ◘ ANSWERS AND RATIONALE

1. **(c)** This patient has had major physiologic stressors and may reasonably anticipate pain for several more weeks. As he makes the transition to prn management, he should be encouraged to take his medication at the onset of pain as this will afford the greatest control. At this point he should not try to push himself to tolerate pain, as it will likely inhibit mobility and prolong recovery. Benzodiazepines are not pain medications and are not routinely used to augment narcotics (Marino, 2007; Tollison, 2002).

2. **(b)** The patient was on a continuous infusion of opioids and benzodiazepines and there may be residual effects from the medications. Prior to ordering other diagnostic tests, mental status can be quickly assessed by reversing those agents. Flumazenil is a benzodiazepine antagonist and can be used to reverse the lorazepam. While residual morphine may be contributing to symptoms, lorazepam has a significantly longer half life and is probably the primary cause of his sedation. If necessary, Narcan may also be given. If mental status does not improve after administration of reversal agents, then diagnostic modalities would be indicated (Katzung, 2009).

3. **(b)** The WHO has a three-step approach to pain control in both acute and chronic scenarios. Narcotics are introduced in step 2, and according to recommendations are always augmented with an adjuvant nonnarcotic drug to provide a synergistic effect that maximizes pain control with the least amount of narcotic. Nonsteroidal anti-inflammatory drugs (NSAIDs) are the most commonly used adjuvant (WHO, 2010).

4. **(d)** While a variety of peripheral factors relative to medical and surgical recovery may contribute to development of congestive heart failure, immobility in itself does not. However, immobility directly increases the risk of venous thrombosis due to stasis of blood in

the veins. Similarly, immobility inhibits deep breathing, which can increase risk for nosocomial pneumonia. Finally, decreased activity inhibits bowel peristalsis, and can lead to development of ileus (Fauci, 2008).

5. **(d)** As a consequence of natural diuresis and fluid shifting, when a previously healthy adult becomes immobile, there will be a transient increase in urinary output for 4–5 days. If bedrest persists, urine output will decline to the lower levels characteristic of bedridden patients (Doherty, 2009).

6. **(a)** This pain is likely due to diabetic neuropathy. Antiepileptic (AED) drugs have the greatest efficacy in neuropathic pain and do not have the same risks of adverse effects and addiction. Antiepileptics and antidepressant medications should be optimized before introducing narcotics for longterm neuropathic pain management. Steroids are not indicated as the pain is not inflammatory, and would actually contribute to ulcer development and poor glycemic control (Tollison, 2002).

7. **(a)** The best approach is to add a Fentanyl patch, as Fentanyl is 80 times more potent than morphine and can provide much stronger pain control. A patch is also easy to use and will provide continuous pain control. While the WHO does advocate NSAID use, severe terminal visceral pain is not optimally managed with morphine and an NSAID, and Fentanyl is the better option. Benzodiazepines may reduce anxiety if it is present, but it is not a pain management drug (Katzung, 2009; Tollison, 2002).

8. **(d)** While immobility can contribute to constipation, the primary problem is the chronic narcotic. The powerful anticholinergic effects of narcotics will slow down the bowel, produce painful constipation, and can lead to ileus. It is a significant problem in patients requiring chronic narcotics, and several medications have been developed to treat it (Doherty, 2009; Katzung, 2009).

9. **(b)** Deconditioning of the baroreceptor reflex in the cardiovascular system can occur within days of bedrest. To avoid this process, avoid bedrest if possible. If it is not possible to avoid bedrest, the patient should be positioned as close to upright as possible several times a day in order to decrease cardiovascular deconditioning. Although sitting the patient on the side of the bed may be helpful, it will not help in maintaining cardiovascular integrity (Fauci, 2008).

10. **(a)** This patient has been in chronic pain for a period of years, so it is likely that the pain, regardless of original etiology, has developed a neuropathic component. AEDs are without the troublesome side-effect profile of opiates and are not addictive. The most appropriate action would be to introduce AEDs, and when a therapeutic dose is achieved, attempt to wean the Lortab down or off. If long-term narcotic therapy is ultimately required, then it will be appropriate to convert to a long acting dose, but that decision will be made after response to AED is evaluated (Tollison, 2002).

11. **(c)** Thrombophilia is a collective term for hereditary disorders that lead to increased clotting. Stasis and clotting tendency are the two primary risk factors for DVT development. Although obesity is a risk factor for DVT, an increased BMI does not necessarily indicate obesity. Liver disease causes a decrease in clotting factors, and so the patient is at greater risk for bleeding than for clotting (Cooper, 2007).

12. **(b)** The main causes for immobility in the elderly include weakness, stiffness, pain, imbalance, or psychiatric problems. Because of the patient's recent

loss, depression is a very strong possibility, and a Geriatric Depression Scale, or some other form of screening for depression, should be done. Dementia is less likely with acute onset, and cranial imaging is not indicated at this point in the evaluation. Zoloft may be an appropriate intervention, but the patient needs to be fully assessed before any treatment is prescribed (McPhee & Papadakis, 2009).

## ◪ REFERENCES

Cooper, D. H., Krainik, A. J., Lubner, S. J., & Reno, H. E. L. (2007). *The Washington manual of medical therapeutics* (32nd ed.). Philadelphia, PA: Lippincott, Williams, & Wilkins.

Doherty, G. (2009). *Current surgical diagnosis and treatment* (13th ed.). New York: McGraw-Hill.

Fauci, A. S., Braunwald, E., Kasper, D. L., Hauser, S. L., Longo, D. L., Jameson, J. L., & Loscalzo, J. (Eds.). (2008). *Harrison's principles of internal medicine* (17th ed.). New York: McGraw-Hill.

Ferri, F. F. (2006). *Practical guide to the care of the medical patient* (7th ed.). Philadelphia, PA: Mosby, Inc.

Katzung, B. G., Masters, S. B., & Trevor, A. J. (Eds.). (2004). *Basic and clinical pharmacology* (11th ed.). New York: McGraw-Hill.

McPhee, S. J., & Papadakis, M. A. (Eds.). (2009). *Current medical diagnosis and treatment* (48th ed.). New York: McGraw-Hill.

Tollison, C. D., Satterthwaite, J. R., & Tollison, J. W. (2002). *Practical pain management* (3rd ed.). Philadelphia, PA: Lippincott, Williams, & Wilkins.

World Health Organization (WHO). Pain relief ladder. Retrieved on December 13, 2009 from http://www.who.int/cancer/palliative/painladder/en/.

# 16

# Patient Education and Nutrition

*Lynn A. Kelso*

## Select one best answer to the following questions.

1. A 55-year-old female is transferred to the trauma unit following a serious motor vehicle accident. She is unresponsive and was intubated in the field. Her son has been notified of her condition and advises you via telephone that she has a living will and that all further diagnostic evaluation and treatment should be stopped. The ACNP tells him that:

   a. He will have to provide a copy of the living will before it can be implemented.
   b. She needs a thorough evaluation to see if her living will is applicable.
   c. The living will is only valid when signed by both patient and legal representative.
   d. You will uphold the patient's wishes and discontinue aggressive actions.

2. You are caring for a 59-year-old male who suffered an acute myocardial infarction (MI) 5 days ago. The patient and his wife have been reading literature, and they understand about diet and exercise, but they do not understand why he cannot return to work. He feels fine, and he will not be paid for his time off. The ACNP should educate them regarding:

   a. Contraindications to driving
   b. The purpose of cardiac medications
   c. Cardiac muscle healing
   d. Cardiac rehabilitation

3. A 63-year-old patient newly diagnosed with diabetes is now admitted through the emergency department for hypoglycemia. He was well controlled on an insulin regimen when discharged from the hospital after his initial diagnosis 1 month ago. While evaluating the patient, the ACNP should do all of the following except:

   a. Discuss with the patient the option to switch to oral antihyperglycemic agents
   b. Have the patient demonstrate his technique for drawing and injecting his insulin
   c. Collect a 72-hour diet and exercise recall
   d. Order blood, urine, and sputum cultures to rule out infection

4. The ACNP is reviewing the home plan of care for a 22-year-old patient being discharged from the hospital with moderate persistent asthma. You know that she correctly understands her instruction if she says:

   a. "I should make an appointment to see my primary care provider if I wake up in the middle of the night more than 2 times a week."
   b. "I do not need to make an appointment if my peak flow is at least 50% of personal best."
   c. "I do not need any medication adjustments as long as I am not using my rescue inhaler on a daily basis."
   d. "I should rinse out my mouth each time I have to use the rescue inhaler so I don't get thrush."

5. The ACNP is counseling an overweight female patient who is 5'5" and 150 lbs. The patient wants to begin a weight loss plan. She has a wedding to attend in 2 months and wants to look her best. The appropriate response is to tell the patient that:

   a. Incorporating moderately intense exercise on a daily basis will likely result in the minimal weight loss that she needs.
   b. A diet and exercise plan that produces a 500 calorie/day deficit is the appropriate approach.
   c. Her weight is within the upper limits of normal for her height and aggressive weight loss is not appropriate.
   d. Her weight loss needs are not significant and can be safely achieved in 1 month.

6. A 21-year-old female being treated for anorexia nervosa is admitted to your service with a syncopal episode. Her laboratory work is significant for a glucose of 51 mg/dL, Na+ 152 mEq/L, and potassium 2.8 mEq/L. The ACNP recognizes that the biggest immediate risk to the patient is:

   a. Level of consciousness changes
   b. Cardiac dysrhythmia
   c. Seizure
   d. Hypoglycemia

7. A patient is started on enteral feedings 72 hours after being admitted following a motorcycle accident. The patient sustained multiple injuries and is currently recovering from surgical repair of a hepatic laceration, pneumothorax, and open fracture of the right humerus. The patient is obese with weight at 275 lbs and height at 5'9". The ACNP knows that his 24-hour caloric intake should be approximately:

   a. 4000 kcal/day
   b. 6000 kcal/day
   c. 8000 kcal/day
   d. 10,000 kcal/day

8. A patient who is being dialyzed for acute renal failure following a 35% full-thickness burn injury is on total enteral nutrition. Morning laboratory studies reveal Na+ 142 mEq/L, K+ 5.3 mEq/L, blood urea nitrogen (BUN) 93 mg/dL, and creatinine 2.1 mg/dL. She has been dialyzed daily with minimal decrease in her BUN. The appropriate action would be to:

   a. Continue to dialyze daily for elevated BUN
   b. Decrease protein intake due to the increased BUN
   c. Place on continuous renal replacement therapy
   d. Change to total parenteral nutrition

9. A 53-year-old female with a 2.5 year history of colon cancer has been on total parenteral nutrition (TPN) at home for 5 months. Her condition is terminal, with death anticipated in a matter of months at best, and while curative care has been aborted, she is still normally awake and alert enough to interact with family. She is admitted to the community hospital for evaluation of increasing somnolence and disorientation. Initial orders should include:

a. Discontinuation of narcotics
b. A head CT scan
c. Liver function studies
d. A psychiatric evaluation

10. When counseling any patient about optimal nutritional intake, the ACNP knows that:

    a. 50–60% of calories should come from carbohydrate.
    b. 50–60% of calories should come from protein.
    c. 50–60% of calories should come from unsaturated fats.
    d. Daily caloric intake should be divided evenly among the three fuel sources.

11. When assessing the nutritional status of a patient, it is important to include:

    a. Morning weight
    b. Fructosamine level
    c. Diet record
    d. Nitrogen balance

12. An 81-year-old male is admitted for treatment of urosepsis. He has become confused and is not eating. His baseline nutritional status is compromised, and he cannot tolerate the combination of no p.o. intake and an infectious process with fever. The ACNP determines that the best method of nutritional supplementation includes:

    a. Peripheral parenteral nutrition (PPN)
    b. Total parenteral nutrition (TPN)
    c. Nasoduodenal feeding
    d. Nasogastric feeding

## ◘ ANSWERS AND RATIONALE

1. **(b)** Living wills come in a variety of forms, but the common aspect is that they are meant to apply when the patient is terminal with no meaningful hope of recovery. In this case, it is too soon to know if that is the case. The living will can only be implemented if the patient is evaluated and deemed applicable. Once her condition is diagnosed as terminal, a copy of the living will should be in the patient's record. It does not need to be approved or signed by the patient's family if it is properly prepared (McPhee & Papadakis, 2009).

2. **(c)** All of these issues may be important topics for patient education, but in order to address their specific knowledge deficit, the ACNP should educate the patient and his wife regarding the course and trajectory of muscle healing. Patients tend to adhere more readily to a prescribed activity regime if they understand the rationale for it. The patient should understand that although he may feel well, the muscle of his heart is recovering from injury, and overuse before proper healing may retard healing and even lead to further injury. Increased activity, such as in the work environment, can lead to increased myocardial workload and sympathetic stimulation that will antagonize optimal healing (Becker, 1976).

3. **(a)** It is important to evaluate for factors that would have contributed to development of hypoglycemia. It is not appropriate to discontinue insulin based upon one episode of hypoglycemia, and presumably insulin was determined to be the best therapeutic option for him at the time of diagnosis. It is important to assess that he is still drawing and injecting insulin properly; while you may assume that he was able to do it correctly at previous hospital discharge, older patients do become confused, and he may have misplaced written instructions, lost the assistance of a friend or family member, or just not wanted to admit that he forgot how to do it. A change in diet and exercise may change insulin requirements and lead to hypoglycemia on his current regimen. Finally, while infection

would normally increase insulin requirements, it may also increase mobilization of exogenous insulin, decrease intake, or in some other way interfere with glucose/insulin balance. Any acute physiologic process should be evaluated (McPhee & Papadakis, 2009).

4. **(a)** Asthma control is acceptable if the patient is having breakthrough symptoms, or requires a rescue inhaler less than 2 times a week. Nocturnal awakening is considered an asthma symptom, and when it happens more than 2 times weekly, the patient needs a medication adjustment. A personal best of 50% is significant bronchospasm, and the patient should be seen; 80% is the acceptable parameter. The goal for rescue inhalers is that they never be used, but less than 2 times a week is acceptable; greater than that requires a medication adjustment. Finally, the patient should rinse after using inhaled corticosteroids, not inhaled beta agonists (NAEPP, 2007).

5. **(b)** At 5'5", this female patient's ideal body weight (IBW) is 125 lbs; it would be 137.5 lbs if she were large boned. Consequently, a 10% weight loss at least is an appropriate goal, and represents a significant weight alteration. Under normal circumstances, safe weight loss should occur at the rate of 1–2 lbs per week. Her goal is 15–25 lbs, so safe weight loss is not possible in one month. The first step is an intake and activity recall. From there, a 3500 kcal/week (500/day) deficit should be incorporated. One pound = 3500 kilocalorie, so a 500/day deficit will produce a 1 lb/week weight loss. Many patients find it easiest to increase caloric burn by 250 kcal/day and decrease intake by 250 kcal/day (McInnis et al., 2003).

6. **(b)** The immediate risk presented is that of cardiac dysrhythmia secondary to hypokalemia. Replenishing potassium is most important. While hypoglycemia may lead to seizure, the blood sugar is not that low. Similarly, hypernatremia may produce level of consciousness changes, but the sodium is not that high. Electrolytes need to be normalized, and a high protein diet introduced. As her metabolic status normalizes, calories may be increased to restore appropriate weight (Cooper, 2007).

7. **(c)** When a patient is undergoing physiologic stress, caloric intake should be calculated to sustain existing body weight, even if the patient is obese. Weight loss strategies should only be implemented if metabolic status and health are otherwise stable. Maintaining current weight requires 30–35 kcal/kg/day. This patient, at 275 lbs, is 125 kg. 125 x 35 kcal = 4375 kcal/day. However, significant physiologic stress doubles caloric need, so while in the acute recovery phase, this amount should be doubled. (Doherty, 2007).

8. **(a)** In patients with high protein requirements, such as those with burn injuries, you are unable to decrease protein intake because of rising BUN levels. The only course of action is to continue to dialyze the patient according to BUN level (Doherty, 2009; Parrillo & Dellinger, 2008).

9. **(c)** Hepatic dysfunction is common in patients on long-term parenteral nutrition. Liver function should be assessed as it may be a treatable cause of symptoms. While the increasing narcotic requirements of terminal cancer patients may be producing the symptoms, they cannot be discontinued. Colon cancers can metastasize to the brain, but this is less likely and less treatable in this patient, so the diagnostic evaluation is not as compelling. A psychiatric cause is less likely at this point in the disease progression. (McPhee & Papadakis, 2009).

10. **(a)** The three nutritional fuel sources are carbohydrates, proteins, and fats. A healthy diet includes 50–60% carbohydrates, up to 30% fats (< 10% saturated), and 0.8 to 1 g/kg of protein daily. Proper weight loss strategies include an overall reduction of calories while maintaining these parameters (McInnis *et al.*, 2003; USPSTF, 2007).

11. **(c)** Nutritional risk factors should be addressed in the history and physical examination. The best way to begin to assess nutritional status is to do a dietary record or a 24-hour dietary recall. Morning weight is more of an indicator of fluid retention than it is nutritional status. Fructosamine levels indicate glycosolated protein and give an indicator of glycemic control over a 2–3 week period, but do not give an indicator of nutrition. Nitrogen balance gives a 24-hour picture of nutritional state and is typically used to evaluate immediate nutrition interventions (Cooper, 2007; Doherty, 2009; McPhee & Papadakis, 2009).

12. **(d)** Supplementing calories should generally be done in the least invasive way possible for patient safety and efficacy. The bowel should only be bypassed when it is not usable, as in obstruction or conditions requiring bowel rest. In this case there is no contraindication for enteral feeds, so the least invasive gut measure should be used. As there are no risk factors for aspiration, a nasal tube terminating in the stomach is appropriate (Ferri, 2008).

## ◻ REFERENCES

Becker, M. H. (1976). *The health belief model and personal health behavior.* Thorofare, NJ: Slack, Inc.

Cooper, D. H., Krainik, A. J., Lubner, S. J., & Reno, H. E. L. (2007). *The Washington manual of medical therapeutics* (32nd ed.). Philadelphia, PA: Lippincott, Williams, & Wilkins.

Doherty, G. (2009). *Current surgical diagnosis and treatment* (13th ed.). New York: McGraw-Hill.

Ferri, F. F. (2006). *Practical guide to the care of the medical patient* (7th ed.). Philadelphia, PA: Mosby, Inc.

McInnis, K. J., Franklin, B. A., & Rippe, J. M. (2003). Counseling for physical activity in overweight and obese patients. *American Family Physician, 67,* 1249–1256, 1266–1268.

McPhee, S. J., & Papadakis, M. A. (Eds.). (2009). *Current medical diagnosis and treatment* (48th ed.). New York: McGraw-Hill.

National Asthma Education and Prevention Program (NAEPP). (2007). *Expert panel report 3: Guidelines for the diagnosis and management of asthma.* Washington, DC: National Institutes of Health.

Parrillo, J., & Dellinger, R. (Eds.). (2008). *Critical care medicine: Principles of diagnosis and management in the adult* (3rd ed.). St. Louis: Mosby, Inc.

# 17

# Psychosocial Issues

*Candis Morrison and Lynn A. Kelso*

## Select one best answer to the following questions.

1. R. S. is a 57-year-old widow of 6 years. Over the course of the past 2 years she has experienced intermittent episodes of anorexia, difficulty sleeping, fatigue, and lethargy. She has to force herself to leave the house to participate in activities that she formerly enjoyed; she just no longer enjoys anything that she does, and does not look forward to any activities. She has no significant medical or surgical history. The physical examination is negative. The most likely diagnosis for this patient is:

   a. Bipolar disorder
   b. Adjustment disorder
   c. Agoraphobia
   d. Major depression

2. Which of the following features differentiates major depressive disorder from a normal grief reaction?

   a. Duration of the symptoms
   b. Severity of the symptoms
   c. Associated vegetative symptoms
   d. History of loss of her spouse

3. A 19-year-old female is brought to the emergency department by her mother. The mother suspects that the daughter is on ecstasy. According to the mother, the patient disappears for a couple of days at a time, and today when she came home she was acting "funny." The ACNP expects which of the following physical findings consistent with ecstasy intoxication?

   a. Overconfidence and teeth grinding
   b. Euphoria and increased appetite
   c. Disinhibition and bradycardia
   d. Disorientation and constricted pupils

4. A 21-year-old male is seen in the urgent care center requesting an HIV test. Night sweats and palpitations have been waking him from sleep for the past 10 days, and he read that these can be symptoms of AIDS. He also admits to getting tightness in his chest, and sometimes his hands get numb. His social history is negative for high-risk sexual behaviors or substance use. Further questioning reveals several stressors; he is living away from home in the dorm. School is not going well, and his

girlfriend just broke up with him. The ACNP suspects that his management will probably include:

a. Propranolol
b. Escitalopram
c. Alprazolam
d. Venlafaxine

5. M. R. is a 42-year-old male patient who is being treated unsuccessfully for depression with serotonin norepinephrine re-uptake inhibitors. He confides to the ACNP that his primary conflict is with his sexuality. He feels that he is really a woman, was born a woman, and wants to have surgery to live his life as a physical woman. The ACNP knows his diagnosis will be best classified as:

a. Transvestism
b. Gender identity disorder
c. Transgenderism
d. Transsexualism

6. W. A., a 32-year-old female, is brought to the emergency department with a fractured right radius and facial ecchymoses. The ACNP notes that her story of tripping and falling into the car door is not consistent with objective findings. Her records reveal that she has had two other extremity fractures, a concussion, and a laceration to the abdomen over the past 3 years. Historical factors that may lead you to suspect domestic violence include:

a. A history of substance abuse in her spouse
b. A spouse > 40 years old
c. A partner of minority cultural background
d. A household income < $35,000 per year

7. A 73-year-old male is admitted for open reduction and internal fixation of a left hip fracture. His wife reports that he has been having "problems" for the last few years, but now his forgetfulness is actually causing him to have little accidents including this fall. During interview he is pleasant and interactive, oriented x 2, with no blatant mental status deficits. The ACNP will refer him for a more thorough evaluation but suspects that the patient has:

a. Delirium
b. Parkinson's disease
c. Depression
d. Dementia

8. The ACNP is performing the initial history and physical examination for a 48-year-old female being treated for ovarian cancer. Overall she feels as though she and her family are coping well. She does admit that she has been feeling depressed for the last few months. She is no longer able to work and has recently been unable to keep up with housework. However, her husband has a good job, and her 14-year-old daughter has been a significant help in managing the household. The patient has been feeling depressed since her activity decreased. While discussing her depression, you ask about:

a. Anger she has toward her husband
b. Guilt she has related to her daughter
c. Fear about her future
d. Denial of her disease process

9. A 42-year-old female has metastatic breast cancer. She remains comfortable on a continuous hydromorphone infusion and is able to minimally participate in activities of daily living (ADL). Her husband is her primary caregiver, and he comes to you to discuss a code status for his wife. With respect to the ethical principles that guide nursing practice, the ACNP tells the husband that:

a. The patient must be involved in the discussion.
b. The topic should be addressed during a palliative care consultation.
c. The attending physician should be consulted.
d. The patient cannot consent to a DNR while on hydromorphone.

10. You are evaluating a 71-year-old male who was recently admitted for pneumonia and an exacerbation of congestive heart failure. He has bilateral below the knee amputations and has been wheelchair-bound for three years. Although he is functional with the assistance of a family friend caregiver at home, he is not acutely incontinent of urine. Since being admitted he has been confused, incontinent, and the caregiver says he now has "Alzheimer's" and that he won't be able to care for him at home anymore. The ACNP explains that:

    a. A social work consult can be ordered to assist with the selection of appropriate long-term care placement.
    b. There are a variety of incontinence aids available to assist with home management.
    c. Acute illness can accelerate an underlying dementia, but that there are a variety of interventions available for management.
    d. The patient is experiencing acute delirium, and that the new symptoms will go away when his pneumonia is treated.

## ◘ ANSWERS AND RATIONALE

1. **(d)** One can make a diagnosis of major depression if five of the nine major depression symptoms are present: Depressed mood, anhedonia (lack of interest or pleasure in all or almost all activities), sleep disorder, appetite change, fatigue or loss of energy, psychomotor retardation or agitation, trouble concentrating or difficulty making decisions, low self-esteem or guilt, recurrent thoughts of death, or suicidal ideation. One of the five must be either depressed mood or anhedonia. There is no suggestion of mania, which is a component of the bipolar diagnoses. There is also no specific stressor or significant social impairment seen with adjustment disorder, and no evidence of phobic behaviors (APA, 2000).

2. **(a)** Grief reaction may include any of the features typically seen in major depressive disorder, and they may be quite severe. The only difference is in the duration of symptoms. DSM-IV-TR indicates that if depressive symptoms are still present 2 months following the loss, the diagnosis of major depressive disorder may be made (APA, 2000; Maercker, 2007).

3. **(a)** Ecstasy is a central nervous system stimulant. Signs and symptoms of intoxication include hyperthermia, tachycardia, hypertension, euphoria, a general feeling of wellness, overconfidence, jaw clenching, teeth grinding, and dilated pupils (McPhee & Papadakis, 2009).

4. **(b)** This young man's presentation is suspicious for generalized anxiety disorder. It is the most common anxiety disorder, and typically appears between 20 and 35 years of age. The disabling anxiety symptoms of apprehension, worry, irritability, hypervigilance, and somatic complaints are present for more than 1 month. Tachycardia, increased BP, epigastric distress, headache, chest tightness and syncope are common symptoms. While benzodiazepines are useful for acute or short-term manifestations, the treatment of choice for control of anxiety disorders is a selective serotonin re-uptake inhibitor (SSRI) (APA, 2000).

5. **(d)** Gender identity disorder is a DSM-IV-TR (and ICD-10) diagnosis code that encompasses several disorders of sexuality. Transsexuality is one type of gender identity disorder in which the patient identifies with the sex opposite the biological one. It is frequently accompanied by the desire to physically alter the body (sexual reassignment surgery) to match the identified gender. Transgenderism is different in that it applies to patients who feel a deviation from normal gender roles; it does not imply a form of sexual orientation.

Transvestites are those who enjoy dressing like the opposite sex; it does not imply a desire to change gender or homosexuality (APA, 2000).

6. **(a)** This is a typical history for a battered woman. Though no well-defined criteria exist to predict who will be battered, some high risk characteristics have been identified: (1) those who are single, divorced, or planning a separation, (2) those between the ages of 17 and 28, (3) those who abuse alcohol or other drugs or whose partners do, (4) those who are pregnant, and (5) those whose partners are excessively jealous or possessive. There are no economic or racial predictors of women at risk (Noble, 2001).

7. **(d)** The progressive and insidious nature of the symptoms suggest a dementing disease, of which Alzheimer's is the most common. Delirium would be much more acute and global in its presentation, depression would exhibit either a depressed mood or anhedonia along with four other symptoms of depression, and Parkinson's disease would present with motor symptoms. Finally, Parkinson's is not primarily a disorder of altered cognition (Wilmoth & Ferraro, 2006).

8. **(b)** Although there is little research on young caregivers of ill adults, the literature does show that parents feel guilty about young or adolescent children becoming their caregivers. Since her depression began at about the time the daughter had to increase her role as caregiver, this is a good area upon which to focus (McPhee & Papadakis, 2009).

9. **(a)** When discussing life-sustaining treatment decisions, the ethical principles that guide nursing practice should be followed. Autonomy (the competent patient's right to make decisions regarding care) requires that the patient be involved in the conversation if able. This patient is minimally participating in her care. Therefore, she must be part of any code status conversation. Narcotics do not prohibit the ability to consent to code status, and while the attending physician will be involved at some point, the initial discussion must include the patient. A palliative care consult will likely be initiated after the patient elects a do-not-resuscitate status (ANA, 2001; Thompson et al., 2006).

10. **(d)** Delirium is a common symptom of infection in the elderly, and his acute and global onset are consistent with delirium rather than dementia. The combination of infection, immobility, and treatment of CHF put him at great risk for transient incontinence. This caregiver needs to be educated that these symptoms are transient and will resolve once the acute processes are controlled (McPhee & Papadakis, 2009).

## ◼ REFERENCES

American Nurses Association (ANA). (2001). *Code of ethics for nurses with interpretive statements.* Silver Spring, MD: Nursesbooks.

American Psychiatric Association (APA). (2000). *Diagnostic and statistical manual of mental disorders* (4th ed., text revision). Washington, DC: Author.

Maercker, A. (2007). When grief becomes a disorder. *European Archives of Psychiatry and Clinical Neuroscience, 257,* 435–436.

McPhee, S. J., & Papadakis, M. A. (Eds.). (2009). *Current medical diagnosis and treatment* (48th ed.), New York: McGraw-Hill.

Noble, J. (2001). *Textbook of primary care medicine* (3rd ed.). St. Louis: Mosby, Inc.

Thompson, I. E., Melia, K. M., Boyd, K. M., & Horsburgh, D. (2006). *Nursing ethics* (5th ed.). London: Churchill Livingstone.

Wilmoth, J., & Ferraro, K. F. (2006). *Gerontology perspectives and issues* (3rd ed.). New York: Springer Publishing Company.

# 18

# Professional Issues and Trends in Advanced Practice

*Ruth M. Kleinpell*

## Select one best answer to the following questions.

1. The ACNP is obtaining informed consent from a 41-year-old patient and is planning an exploratory laparotomy for recurrent abdominal pain. The consent includes a paragraph authorizing blood transfusions if needed. The patient says, "I am a Jehovah's Witness and we do not believe in transfusions. I will not consent to a blood transfusion." The appropriate action by the ACNP would be to:

   a. Counsel the patient that the procedure carries a significant risk of blood loss and that she cannot have the procedure without consenting

   b. Honor the patient's preferences, counsel her about the risks of refusing blood transfusion, discuss alternatives, and be sure that everything is well documented

   c. Suggest that she consider banking her own blood preoperatively in the event that her blood loss requires transfusion

   d. Consult the unit social worker to seek advice on obtaining a court-ordered consent

2. While preparing to establish a therapeutic relationship with a new patient, the ACNP begins by:

   a. Assessing his own feelings, fears, and anxieties

   b. Establishing trust and sharing information with the patient

   c. Setting goals with the patient for therapeutic outcomes

   d. Helping the patient identify anxieties and develop coping skills

3. Mrs. W. is an 84-year-old female who was admitted for management of community-acquired pneumonia. She is remarkably strong, and a positive outcome is anticipated. However, as part of routine admission procedure she is offered the opportunity to sign a living will. She asks if the living will is legal, and whether or not her son can overturn it if she becomes unable to communicate. The best answer is to tell her that:

a. In accordance with the Patient Self-Determination Act of 1990, living wills signed by a competent patient at the time of admission are legally binding.

b. While it is technically legally binding, it would be best to obtain her son's signature also if she anticipates any conflict.

c. Living wills are not legally binding and are meant to be a written expression of wishes that are generally followed if there is no familial conflict.

d. Not all advanced directives are legally binding, and that if she wants to be sure hers is, she should consult with an attorney.

4. Privacy and confidentiality are important components of patients' rights, and the ACNP should understand elements of both. Which of the following is not an accurate statement regarding privacy and confidentiality?

a. When there is a conflict between privacy and confidentiality, confidentiality is the priority.

b. The patient's right to privacy guarantees that he can be sure that his health information will be shared only with those involved in his care.

c. Protecting confidentiality includes protecting the use of identifying information.

d. Placing a patient in a public position in a false light is a violation of privacy.

5. The ACNP is now eligible for Medicare reimbursement. Reimbursement of NP services to Medicare patients:

a. Can vary from state to state

b. Consists of part A covering outpatient care and part B covering inpatient care

c. Requires the NP to work in collaboration with a physician in some states

d. Allows direct NP reimbursement in some settings

6. The ACNP is providing discharge teaching to a 54-year-old female patient who was admitted for treatment of complicated pyelonephritis. She has recovered nicely and is preparing to go home. The ACNP knows that discharge teaching should include:

a. A review of genitourinary hygiene to decrease risk for reinfection

b. A reminder that she should ensure that her mammogram, lipid, and colon cancer screenings are current

c. Information on annual influenza and pneumococcal vaccination indication and availability

d. Counseling about always wearing her seat belt while driving

7. Ruth T. has been hired as an ACNP to work with a group of cardiologists. Her role will incorporate both inpatient care and outpatient clinic responsibilities. Her ACNP position:

a. Will require her to obtain credentialing privileges for hospital practice

b. Will encompass substitutive care traditionally given by physicians

c. Is considered to be a service-based practice model

d. Must be supervised by a physician in the inpatient setting

8. Who among the following represents the leading cause of cancer mortality in the United States?

a. A 57-year-old male with stage IV prostate cancer

b. A 43-year-old female with stage III colon cancer

c. A 51-year-old female with breast cancer

d. A 72-year-old male with lung cancer

9. Evidence-based practice is the goal for healthcare provision in the US and should be the foundation for acute care nurse practitioner practice. All of the following are standards of evidence-based practice except:

a. Patching the affected eye for 24 hours in corneal abrasion

b. Prescribing azithromycin for community-acquired pneumonia in an otherwise healthy patient

c. Diagnosing blood pressure based upon > 2 readings on 2 or more occasions

d. Using amoxicillin as a first-line drug therapy for sinusitis

10. Jason J. is a newly certified and licensed ACNP and is interviewing for positions. While interviewing at a major tertiary care facility, he is informed that claims-made malpractice insurance coverage is included as part of the compensation package. This means that he:

a. Should be protected for any claim made relative to an incident that occurred when he was working there

b. Would be best protected to purchase his own occurrence-based policy

c. Will need to consider tail coverage at some point

d. Should request a copy of the policy showing his name added to the list of insured providers

11. In accordance with current standards of practice, the ACNP knows that a hypertensive urgency should be treated with:

a. Sublingual nifedipine

b. Intravenous vasodilators

c. Any short acting oral agent used to treat hypertension

d. A thiazide diuretic/beta blocker combination

12. According to American Heart Association and the American College of Sports Medicine, current recommendations for exercise for all adults include:

a. Resistance training at least two times weekly

b. Moderate activity for 30 minutes 3 to 5 times weekly

c. A complete history and physical exam before starting a program

d. An assessment of blood pressure and fractionated cholesterol before beginning

13. Patients who are immobile and subject to bedrest for extended periods of time are at increased risk for decubitus ulcer formation. The ACNP knows that leading risk factors for decubitus development include all of the following except:

a. Prolonged friction

b. Shear forces

c. Nutritional debilitation

d. High blood pressure

14. A 62-year-old patient is having persistent lower extremity pain as a result of poorly controlled type 2 diabetes. While considering treatment options for neuropathic pain, the ACNP knows that common adverse effects of tricyclic antidepressants include all of the following except:

a. Diarrhea

b. Urinary retention

c. Cardiac dysrhythmia

d. Sedation

15. According to current evidence, the ACNP knows that risk of cardiovascular complications is markedly decreased in a patient when:

a. Blood pressure is maintained < 120/80 mm Hg

b. Fasting blood sugar is maintained < 126 mg/dL

c. Total cholesterol is maintained < 200 mg/dL

d. Hemoglobin is maintained < 13 g/dL

16. Which of the following statements best reflects current evidence-based information about cancer risk?

a. Risk of cervical cancer is not increased by family history

b. Risk of lung cancer is not increased by family history

c. Family history of virtually any cancer increases risk

d. Obesity increases risk for prostate cancer

17. Research can be categorized as experimental and nonexperimental. Nonexperimental research:

    a. Is the strongest type of research design for a study
    b. Involves manipulation of variables but lacks a control group
    c. Describes or examines relationships among variables
    d. Tests the effects of an intervention or experiment

18. A variety of theories are postulated to drive healthcare-related beliefs and behaviors. While counseling a patient about the importance of smoking cessation, the ACNP finds that the patient already recognizes the need and has designed for himself a "stop-smoking" plan according to which he will smoke his last cigarette 30 days from today. The ACNP knows that this represents which stage of the transtheoretical model of change?

    a. Precontemplation
    b. Contemplation
    c. Preparation
    d. Action

19. Which of the following is not a goal statement in *Healthy People 2020*?

    a. Attain high quality, longer lives free of preventable disease, disability, injury, and premature death
    b. Achieve health equity, eliminate disparities, and improve the health of all groups
    c. Increase the proportion of persons who receive appropriate evidence-based clinical preventive services
    d. Create social and physical environments that promote good health for all

20. Performance of a routine mammogram represents which level of prevention?

    a. Primary
    b. Secondary
    c. Tertiary
    d. Rehabilitative

21. Mrs. W. is a 75-year-old patient who suffered a cerebral infarct 2 weeks ago. After a turbulent hospital course, she is finally ready for discharge. The ACNP has referred Mrs. W. to an inpatient rehabilitation facility. This is an example of which level of health prevention?

    a. Primary
    b. Secondary
    c. Tertiary
    d. Rehabilitative

22. The ACNP is advising an uninsured 57-year old patient on how to access health care. The patient has heard of Medicare and Medicaid but doesn't understand the difference between the two. The ACNP knows that which of the following is a true statement with regard to Medicaid?

    a. It is a federally funded and administered health program
    b. It is a state funded and administered health program
    c. It is a government-sponsored supplemental medical insurance
    d. It is a federally supported, state administered health program

23. Kevin is a service-based ACNP who is managing all patients admitted to the internal medicine service. A patient is transferred to his care who has a variety of medical conditions and is deteriorating fairly quickly. Kevin reviews the patient's chart for the presence of an advance directive. This is because he knows that The Patient Self-Determination Act of 1990 requires that all patients have the right to:

    a. Designate level of care
    b. Designate a legal guardian
    c. Designate a power of attorney
    d. Designate end-of-life care choices

24. The ACNP is planning to obtain informed consent for a central line insertion. In order to give informed consent, the patient must be able to understand all of the following except:

    a. The nature and purpose of the procedure
    b. The benefits, risks, and adverse effects
    c. Reasonable alternatives
    d. Anticipated costs

25. A 66-year-old female patient in the intensive care unit has reached an end stage of a variety of medical conditions including multiple sclerosis. She is currently bedridden with a limited quality of life, and has decided that she does not want any more interventions with the exception of comfort care. Later in the day her mental status begins to deteriorate, and the service resident wants to perform a CT scan of her head. The patient does not understand how a CT scan will improve her comfort care and wants to know why the scan should be performed. In explaining that the CT scan will not impact comfort care, the ACNP is exercising her ethical duty of:

    a. Autonomy
    b. Veracity
    c. Beneficence
    d. Justice

26. Patient education is an important part of holistic care, and often is supplemented with written materials that the patient can take home and review. When providing patient education materials, the ACNP remembers that:

    a. The average adult reading level is eighth to ninth grade.
    b. Black is the easiest color to see for those who may have eye conditions.
    c. Written materials have not demonstrated any increase in patient understanding.
    d. Written materials are more effective than verbal instruction.

27. A potential employer is interviewing an ACNP candidate for a position in a different state and asks the candidate whether or not she is able to prescribe narcotic analgesics. The ACNP candidate replies:

    a. Prescriptive practice is state-specific, and we need to review your state's practice act.
    b. Nurse practitioners are authorized to have DEA numbers and are legally authorized to prescribe.
    c. Nurse practitioners are authorized to have DEA numbers and may prescribe in inpatient settings if allowed by the institution.
    d. Narcotic prescribing is permissible in the inpatient setting as long as there is a collaborative physician.

28. The American Nurses Association's Scope and Standards of Practice for the Acute Care Nurse Practitioner identifies all of the following as essential roles for acute care nurse practitioners except for:

    a. Clinician
    b. Consultant
    c. Collaborator
    d. Leader

29. The ACNP is a member of a committee working on a quality improvement initiative to better structure care after open heart surgery, including when vital signs, laboratory and diagnostic tests, and aspects of care are to be completed. This is an example of:

    a. Quality planning
    b. Diagnosis related group (DRG) care
    c. Developing a critical pathway
    d. Multidisciplinary care

30. Many states require that nurse practitioners be certified as a condition of state licensure. The ACNP knows that the primary difference between licensure and certification is that:

    a. Licensure is a government-mandated requirement to practice
    b. Certification is a nongovernment-mandated requirement to practice

c. Licensure is required to prescribe narcotics
d. Certification is required in states with independent practice

31. While preparing for the ACNP certification exam, J. H. is reviewing the ethical principles of nursing practice. He remembers that the ethical principle of veracity represents the duty of the nurse practitioner to:

a. Do the greatest good
b. Do no harm
c. Be truthful
d. Be fair

32. A newly hired ACNP negotiates for malpractice insurance coverage as part of her employment benefits. Malpractice insurance:

a. Will protect the ACNP from charges related to invasive procedural work traditionally performed by a physician
b. Will only protect the ACNP from charges related to injury to the patient
c. Will not protect the ACNP from charges of practicing medicine without a license if practicing outside the legal scope of practice for the state
d. Will protect the ACNP from charges of practicing medicine without a license as long as clinical privileges have been obtained

33. J. R. is a 66-year-old female with terminal cervical cancer. While considering her options, she is trying to balance cost with benefit. She wants to pursue hospice care, but is afraid she cannot afford it. The ACNP advises her that Medicare part A covers all of the following except:

a. Short-term skilled nursing facility care
b. Hospice care
c. Home health agency visits
d. Outpatient hospital care

34. An ACNP is employed by a managed care network to practice in a multi-practice clinic. Which of the following is accurate regarding managed care networks?

a. They contractually agree to provide services for certain patient groups.
b. They usually allow the patient to choose a provider and/or hospital for a minimal copay.
c. They are funded with a fixed percentage of federal dollars.
d. The model of care emphasizes case coordination.

35. While interviewing for a position as an ACNP with a group of cardiologists, the physician asks the ACNP about billing procedures. The NP will be assigned to the hospital patients, and will be doing all new cardiology consults. It is the physician's plan to bill for the NP services as "incident to" so that the services provided by the ACNP are reimbursed at 100% of the physician rate. The ACNP tells him that:

a. The physician must be physically present in the facility when the ACNP renders the service in order to bill "incident to."
b. "Incident to" billing cannot be used to bill for inpatient services under any circumstances.
c. "Incident to" billing cannot be used for new consults, only for care of existing hospital patients.
d. The physician must be immediately available by electronic means when the ACNP renders the service in order to bill "incident to."

36. J. R. is an ACNP who is beginning to explore independent practice opportunities. While developing a business plan, she investigates sources and mechanisms of reimbursement. She finds that she may be reimbursed nationally through which of the following programs?

a. CHAMPUS
b. Private insurance companies

c. Managed care networks

d. Social Security Administration

37. Preferred Provider Organizations (PPOs) are:

a. Fee-for-service provider partnerships

b. A type of HMO

c. A type of managed care system

d. An HMO subplan

38. Which of the following is accurate regarding the National Practitioner Data Bank?

a. It is a professional registry for advanced practice nurses.

b. It is a governmental resource of current legislation pertinent to nurse practitioner practice.

c. It provides voluntary listings for physicians and advanced practice nurses by professional area of expertise.

d. It compiles information on medical-legal actions taken against health-care professionals.

## ☐ ANSWERS AND RATIONALE

1. **(b)** Cultural and religious sensitivity is an essential part of the nurse practitioner–patient relationship. Competent patients have the right to determine their own care, and this patient has the right to refuse consent. The only option is to present all alternatives, inform as to increased risk, and document the interaction well. The Jehovah's Witnesses governing body has ruled out the use of preoperative blood banking (ANA, 2001).

2. **(a)** The therapeutic relationship should begin with a pre-orientation phase in which the ACNP identifies his own feelings, anxieties, and fears before entering the relationship. The orientation phase begins interaction with the patient and includes establishing trust and information sharing. The working phase is where the therapeutic goals are set and met, and the termination phase is the end of that part of the relationship (APA, 2000).

3. **(d)** The legality of living wills and other forms of advanced directives is an ongoing topic of controversy among caregivers and institutions. Generally, when there is no disagreement among family and providers, they are followed without incident. However, when there is a conflict among any of the principles (family, providers, or administrators), the subject of "legality" is often debated. The best response to this patient is that if she anticipates any conflict and wants to ensure a legally binding living will to the best of her ability, she should consult an attorney to draft and sign a legally binding document (USLWR, 2010).

4. **(d)** Violations of privacy include using the patient's name or identifiable part without permission, unreasonable intrusion when there is a right to expect privacy, public disclosure of private facts, and placing the patient publicly in a false light. Confidentiality protects the sharing of information. They are both patient rights, and one is not prioritized over the other (ANA, 2004).

5. **(c)** Medicare is a federally funded health program with part A covering inpatient hospital and posthospital skilled nursing care, home health, and hospice. Part B is a supplemental medical insurance that covers physician visits, outpatient care, home care, laboratory, radiology, and other related medical services and supplies. Direct Medicare reimbursement can be obtained for NP services provided in both rural and urban settings at 85% of physician reimbursement for services provided in collaboration with a physician (Mason et al., 2007).

6. **(b)** At this patient's age her leading risk factors for morbidity and mortality are cancer and vascular disease, so patient education should prioritize these.

Genitourinary hygiene may be helpful as lower urinary infection can increase risk of upper urinary infection, and seat belt use is always important, but she is at greatest risk for death from vascular disease or cancer. Influenza vaccinations are indicated annually but pneumococcal vaccination is not (USPSTF, 2007).

7.  **(c)** ACNP practice models include service-based, practice-based, and population-based practice models. Service-based ACNPs are involved with clinical management of specific patients followed by a medical or surgical group such as surgical oncology or neurology. Practice-based ACNPs are involved with clinical management of patients seen on a particular hospital unit or clinic setting, such as vascular surgery patients. Population-based ACNPs are involved with patients with specific disease entities, such as diabetes. Hospital credentialing and privileging may be required for ACNP practice in the hospital setting. Those privileges would also stipulate the degree of direct supervision required. ACNP practice is not substitutive for physician care, but rather is a comprehensive collaborative care model (Kleinpell, 2005).

8.  **(d)** The leading cause of cancer morbidity and mortality in the US is lung cancer in both genders. Breast cancer is the leading cause of cancer morbidity in women, and prostate the leading cause of cancer morbidity in men. Colon cancer is the third leading cause of cancer morbidity and mortality in both genders (USPSTF, 2007).

9.  **(a)** Evidence-based practice in general terms refers to the use of current evidence in designing assessment and management strategies for patients. Evidence exists on a variety of levels, from empirical research to expert consensus. Current evidence is that patching the eye is not useful, yet many providers continue to do so as it has been a long-standing intervention. Conversely, azithromycin is indicated according the most recent ATS/IDSA guidelines for management of community-acquired pneumonia, three blood pressure readings on two separate occasions is required for diagnosis of HTN according to the Joint National Committee's 7th report, and the Sinus and Allergy Health Partnership (SAHP) guidelines advocate amoxicillin as a first-line approach to sinusitis (JNC, 2004; Polit & Beck, 2008).

10. **(c)** Claims-made coverage only protects if the practitioner has the policy when the claim is made; therefore, anyone covered by a claims-made policy needs to consider tail coverage to protect the provider from the time period between the end of the claims-made policy and the statute of limitations in the individual state. Occurrence-based malpractice insurance protects against any incident that occurred during the time the policy was in effect even if the claim is made when the policy is no longer in effect, and is another option, but the decision between the two is based on a variety of features (Fitzgerald, 2005).

11. **(c)** In accordance with the current standards of care for the assessment and treatment of hypertension, a hypertensive urgency is defined as any condition of upper level stage 2 hypertension or hypertension in the setting of progressive target organ damage. The recommended treatment is the use of any oral agent indicated for the treatment of high blood pressure. Sublingual nifedipine is specifically prohibited by the JNC 7 report (JNC, 2004).

12. **(a)** Current evidence-based recommendations for exercise for adults states that exercise programs should include moderately intense exercise for 30 minutes at least 5 times weekly or

vigorous exercise for 20 minutes 2 times weekly, along with resistance training at least 2 times weekly. A history and physical exam with exercise ECG is recommended when beginning a program after the age of 40 (USPSTS, 2007).

13. **(d)** Leading risk factors for pressure ulcer development are friction, shear forces, and nutritional debilitation. Other contributing factors include moisture, advanced age, low blood pressure, smoking, elevated body temperature, and dehydration (Revis, 2009).

14. **(a)** Tricyclic antidepressants are an effective intervention for neuropathic pain, but are limited by their powerful anticholinergic effects. Anticholinergic effects include sedation, dry mouth, cardiac dysrhythmia, urinary retention, and constipation (Tollison, 2002).

15. **(a)** The JNC 7 report reports evidence that the risk of vascular disease increases when blood pressure rises beyond 120/80 mm Hg, which is why the "prehypertension" category was developed. American diabetes guidelines for blood sugar management suggests that optimal vascular health is maintained when fasting blood sugar is less than 100 mg/dL. While total cholesterol is an acceptable screening mechanism in low-risk patients, a total cholesterol of less than 200 mg/dL does not necessarily mean decreased risk; a fractionated cholesterol level must be assessed. Hemoglobin of less than 13 g/dL does not confer increased vascular risk. (JNC, 2004; NCEP, 2002).

16. **(c)** Even those cancers more commonly associated with environmental exposures, such as cervical and lung, are increased in patients with a family history. This is probably due to a genetic predisposition to respond to carcinogens. Obesity is a risk factor for a variety of cancers, but of more than 35 studies evaluating obesity and prostate cancer, no association has been identified (USPSTF, 2007).

17. **(c)** Nonexperimental research aims to describe situations and experiences or examine relationships among variables. Experimental research has a control group and involves manipulation of a variable, and is considered a stronger research methodology. (Polit & Hungler, 2008).

18. **(b)** The precontemplation stage is characterized by no plans to make the change. The contemplation change includes plans to change behavior within 6 months. The action stage means that overt action that can impact disease has already been taken (Burbank & Riebe, 2001).

19. **(c)** *Healthy People 2020* includes four overarching goals and then a variety of objectives within specific topics. Options "a," "b," and "d" are three of the four goal statements; choice "c" represents one of the many objectives (USDHHS, 2009).

20. **(b)** Performance of a routine mammogram is considered secondary health prevention as it screens for asymptomatic disease before illness occurs. Primary prevention includes those life style strategies used to decrease risk for disease, such as healthy diet, avoiding drugs and alcohol, and safe sex practices. Tertiary prevention entails minimizing existing disease, such as controlling blood pressure or blood sugar in those patients with hypertension or diabetes, or cardiac rehabilitation after myocardial infarction. Rehabilitation is a feature of tertiary prevention (USPSTF, 2009).

21. **(c)** As described in rationale for question #20 above, stroke rehabilitation is considered to be tertiary health prevention (ANA, 2004; Burbank & Riebe, 2002).

22. **(d)** Medicaid is generally regarded as a state-based program, but it is a federally supported, state administered health program for low-income families and individuals. Medicare is a federally funded and administered program for the elderly and those with very specific health conditions, such as dialysis-dependent renal failure (Mason *et al.*, 2007).

23. **(a)** The Patient Self-Determination Act of 1990 requires that all patients have the right to execute an advanced directive. Under the act, at the time of admission healthcare institutions must provide the patient with a written summary of patient healthcare decision-making rights, and advise the patient of the facility's policy in recognizing advanced directives. The act also requires that the facility ask if the patient has an advanced directive, and allow the patient to include it as part of the medical record. It prohibits discrimination against those regardless of advanced directive status, and prohibits the institution from requiring one (Mason *et al.*, 2007).

24. **(d)** Patient competency implies that the patient is able to understand his diagnosis; risks, benefits, and adverse effects; nature and diagnosis of procedure. The patient must also have knowledge of the diagnosis (ANA, 2001; Bell, 2008; Mason *et al.*, 2007).

25. **(b)** The ethical principle of veracity is the duty to be truthful with the patient. Autonomy is the patient's right to determine care; justice is the duty to see that the patient has the opportunities that he deserves; and beneficence is the duty to do the greatest good (ANA, 2001).

26. **(a)** The average adult reading level is eighth to ninth grade. Written materials are an important and helpful supplement to, but not a good substitute for, verbal interaction and instruction.

Multiple colors may actually be more eye-catching and contribute to interest and retention (NCES, 2002).

27. **(a)** Specific practice rights and privileges are always state-specific. Whether or not a nurse practitioner may prescribe at all, or pronounce patients dead, sign a commercial driver's license exam, or any other of a variety of actions is dictated by the state practice act. The drug enforcement agency (DEA) is a federal registry that maintains a registration of those advanced practice nurses authorized by the individual states to prescribe. Every state has different legislation, and some do not require a collaborating physician (Bell, 2008; Joel, 2006).

28. **(d)** The *Scope and Standards of Practice for Acute Care Nurse Practitioners* outlines five roles for ACNPs: Clinician, researcher, collaborator, consultant, and educator. They are all considered equally important (Bell, 2008).

29. **(c)** A critical pathway contains key patient care activities and time for those activities that are needed for a specific-case type of diagnosis related group (DRG). Critical pathways are a blueprint for planning and managing care delivered by all disciplines (Joel, 2006).

30. **(a)** Licensure is required to legally practice in any state and is issued by the state government. Certification is conferred by several nongovernmental boards, and while many states require it as a condition to practice, some do not. Certification does not confer any practice or prescribing privilege in any state, and while an acute care nurse practitioner may or may not be certified depending upon state law, all practicing practitioners must be licensed (ANA, 2004).

31. **(c)** Doing no harm is the ethical principle of nonmalfeasance. Doing the greatest good is the principle of

beneficence, and being truthful embodies the principle of veracity. While being fair is certainly ethical, it is not among the five ethical principles of nursing practice (ANA, 2001).

32. **(c)** Malpractice insurance for the ACNP will not protect the ACNP from charges of practicing medicine without a license if practicing outside the legal scope of practice for the state (Mason *et al.*, 2007).

33. **(d)** Medicare part A covers inpatient care, skilled nursing facilities, hospice care, long-term care, inpatient rehab, home health care, and obesity bariatric surgery. Medicare part B, a supplemental medical insurance, covers outpatient hospital care, physician visits, home care, laboratory, radiology, and other related services (Mason *et al.*, 2007).

34. **(a)** Managed care networks contractually agree to provide services for certain patient groups. They do have a fixed network of providers and facilities, and consumers are not offered a choice. Managed care networks are not federally funded, and do not reimburse providers individually (Mason *et al.*, 2007).

35. **(b)** Medicare rules for "incident to" billing are very specific, and many other insurers follow Medicare rules. Reimbursement of services of nurse practitioners performed "incident-to" physician services means that the nurse practitioner was able to perform services ordinarily performed by the physician. "Incident to" billing cannot be used for new patients, must be in a defined office-suite, and cannot be used in the inpatient setting (Mason *et al.*, 2007).

36. **(a)** Nurse practitioners can be reimbursed nationally through CHAMPUS (Civilian Health and Medical Program of the United Services and FEHBP (Federal Employees Health Benefit Program).

Managed care networks and private insurers are clearly not a mechanism for federal dollars. The Social Security Administration is a federal organization, but does not reimburse providers (Joel, 2006; Mason *et al.*, 2007).

37. **(c)** Preferred provider organizations are a type of managed care system. A partnership is established between a group of "preferred providers" and an insurance company or entity to provide specific medical and hospital care at prearranged costs (Mason *et al.*, 2007).

38. **(d)** The National Practitioner Data Bank, a federal entity, compiles information on medical–legal actions taken against healthcare professionals. Conditions that must be reported include malpractice settlements and adverse actions that influence clinical privileges or licensure. Hospitals are required to query the National Practitioner Data Bank when a provider makes an application for staff or clinical privilege appointments and then every 2 years thereafter (Mason *et al.*, 2007).

# ◘ REFERENCES

American Nurses Association (ANA). (2001). *Code of ethics for nurses with interpretive statements.* Silver Spring, MD: Nursesbooks.

American Nurses Association (ANA). (2004). *Nursing: Scope and standards of practice.* Silver Spring, MD: Nursesbooks.

American Psychiatric Association (APA). (2000). *Diagnostic and statistical manual of mental disorders* (4th ed., text revision). Washington, DC: Author.

Bell, L. (Ed.). (2008). *AACN scope and standards for acute and critical care nursing practice.* Aliso Viejo, CA: American Association of Critical-Care Nurses.

Burbank, P. M., & Riebe, D. (2002). *Promoting exercise and behavior change in older adults: Interventions with the transtheoretical model.* New York: Springer Publishing Company.

Fitzgerald, M. A. (2005). *Nurse practitioner certification and practice preparation guide* (2nd ed.). Philadelphia, PA: F. A. Davis.

Joel, L. A. (2009). *Advanced practice nursing: Essentials for role development* (2nd ed.). Philadelphia, PA: F. A. Davis.

Joint National Committee on Prevention, Detection, Evaluation, and Treatment of High Blood Pressure (JNC). (2004). *7th report of the JNC.* Washington, DC: National Institutes of Health (update due Summer 2010).

Kleinpell, R. M. (2005). Acute care nurse practitioner practice: Results of a 5-year longitudinal study. *American Journal of Critical Care, 14,* 211–219.

Mason, D. J., Leavitt, J. K., & Chaffee, M. W. (2007). *Policy and politics in nursing and health care* (5th ed.). Philadelphia, PA: Saunders.

National Center for Education Statistics (NCES). (2002). *Adult literacy in America (NALS).* Washington, DC: Author.

National Cholesterol Education Panel (NCEP). (2002). *Third report of the expert panel on detection, evaluation, and treatment of high blood cholesterol in adults (Adult Treatment Panel III).* Washington, DC: National Institutes of Health (update due Summer 2010).

Polit, D. F., & Beck, C. T. (2008). *Nursing research: Generating and assessing evidence for nursing practice* (8th ed.). Philadelphia, PA: Lippincott, Williams, & Wilkins.

Revis, D. R. (2005). Decubitus ulcers. *Emedicine.* Retrieved April 29, 2007 from www.emedicine.com/med/topic2709.htm.

Tollison, C. D., Satterthwaite, J. R., & Tollison, J. W. (2002). *Practical pain management.* (3rd ed.). Philadelphia, PA: Lippincott, Williams, & Wilkins.

US Living Will Registry (USLWR). (2010). Retrieved January 13, 2010 from http://www.uslivingwillregistry.com/.

United States Department of Health and Human Services (USDHHS). (2009). *Healthy people 2020 framework.* Washington, DC: Author.

# Index